The ~~Secret~~ Diaries of

Menopausal Women

A book on feeling good when you REALLY feel bad.

Jacqueline Golding

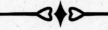

Acknowledgements

I would like to, first and foremost, thank the creator of life. For with life, all things are possible.

To my children, who have supported me entirely on this new and challenging journey, but particularly for always believing in my power, even when I forgot how truly powerful I am. Even as a writer, there are not enough words to describe the immense love that I have for you both.

Thank you to my brother, Michael, for editing this masterpiece in a timely fashion. I know you chose to lead a laid-back, peaceful life, so, for your speed and thoroughness, I am forever grateful. More importantly, I thank you for being there for that scared little girl back then, and for the little girl still with me today. For always believing in me, I'm truly thankful.

Thank you, with all my heart, to both Fiona and Roshan, for support with the first and third edits of this book. Your insight and humour have helped me to get to the end of this emotional journey in one piece.

To my daddy, who has always been the constant love in my life. I could not have ever asked for more from you, you are my guiding light on all of my dark days.

To my mum, for all that we could not be for each other, I'm sorry. For all that we have been for each other, I am grateful. I love you.

Thank you to my cousin Sarah, for everything. I truly appreciate our sisterhood and friendship and obviously my amazing hair.

A huge amount of appreciation to Courtney Freckleton, my PA, who has supported me and stuck by me, even on my darkest days, always with the biggest smile that encapsulates my heart every day. Thank you for sharing my joy, my tears, my fears and my laughter.

Thank you to Angela, for all your beautiful creative insight and beautiful spirit. This has helped me to stay grounded.

To the amazing ladies who chose me to share their journeys with, I am eternally honoured and privileged for being trusted with the most private parts of your life; Charlie Jenkins, Karen Keohone, Averil MacGillivray, Caterina Gatenby, Lisa Gair, Lynsey Ashworth, Carol Sorhaindo, Nicola Jane Gifford, Karen Miller, Sara Meekley, Annie Hayes-Pantony, Phyllis Woodly, Mastaneh Azizi Babany, Jo-Ann Eisenberg, Alicia Mulholland, Barbara Burchell, Fiona Maida, Gillian Shipley, Sara Gilmartin, Ama Owusua, Jayne Pick, Christina Decillo, Sally Cork, Tithi Ghosh, Rehana Malik, Natasha Logan and Margie De Sousa. Thank you, from the bottom of my heart. I am sure that your stories will help millions of women to feel whole again. We all know that it is not easy, but we know that together, as Sisters, we can make it!!

Lastly, thank you to my readers, if you are here then we are now sisters.

I wish you love and light on your life journey, whatever you are going through, and I look forward to your evolution. Stay mindful, stay in peace, but most of all, remember that together, we are stronger.

One Love, walk tall and be blessed.

A Woman's World

A poem by Jacqueline Golding

It's a woman's world, of this I'm sure

No one else this life so fearless could endure,

A woman just knows she sews; she flows, loves, heals, tends, and glows.

With the heart of a lion, the soul of an angel

There's always an extra seat at her table.

Strength all the way from her head to her feet,

Her manner can present both bitter and sweet.

A woman determined and triumphant

I am that woman!!

What a woman!!

That's me.

Dedication

With love, I dedicate this book to my 3.9 billion sisters across the globe.

May these stories give you some comfort and understanding.

May they strengthen your resilience and renew your hope.

One Love

Contents

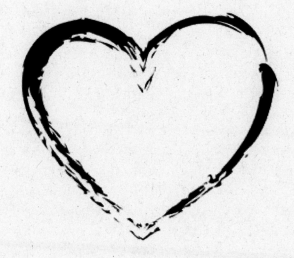

Introduction

Had anybody ever told me that I would feel as though I could "literally" murder somebody one day, I would have told them they were crazy.

Fast forward to the ripe old age of forty-four, and I reach the point in my life when the above statement is true. Due to the fact that nobody has prepared me for the massive number of changes that my body starts to endure, my mind struggles to connect the dots as I sink deeper and deeper into a confused state of "craziness".

One of the many things I have learned on my menopausal journey is that very few women are taught about this stage of their life. First the perimenopause, then the menopause and into post-menopause. Through this lack of awareness, the many changes that we face can mean that it often comes like a thief in the night, taking with it your sanity, your independence and your physical well-being. At times, causing mass confusion with your family and friends, turning your life upside down, shaking you, breaking you and then finally "making you".

Hence this diary, to share my journey with those who have travelled before me, with me and for those yet to travel.

When I think of a diary, I think of the passage of time, the plotting of new ventures, memories of raising children and relationship goals. I also think of keeping up with work commitments, pursuing hobbies and building dreams. I wanted to mark this challenging phase of my life with a vibrant diary of my experiences. I want to exclaim that I survived and lived to tell the tale, as sadly, some do not.

Compiling a collective diary with other women came to me as a divine afterthought.

Why do I think this?

Well, I have always been known to speak my mind, often being the topic of many dinner table talks. On my journey through life and way before this menopause stage, I had stopped allowing others to use their words to define me. Instead, I started to cherish the gifts bestowed upon me, gifts of confidence and speech. My motto has long been, "you may love me, you may hate me, but I have a gift to walk where angels fear to tread". My gifts have always been a dash of courage, with a splash of words, topped off with a sprinkle of deep emotional insight.

Ten years ago, I learned that I was an empath... a person who feels things deeply. Sometimes so deeply that it can affect your state of peace. The Oxford dictionary states that an empath is "a person with the paranormal ability to perceive the mental or emotional state of another individual".

My gifts have helped me speak for those who cannot always speak for themselves. It is with great pride and sensitivity that I am using them to provide a vessel for the voiceless and a funnel for the future queens fighting this taboo subject for the greater good.

I was armed with this knowledge so this is when my idea evolved. I interviewed many women from many different walks of life for this project and listened to each story. I heard many unspoken words behind every pair of eyes, as I looked deep into their souls. Intertwined personal journeys of women from around the world, compiled in a sometimes humorous but always sensitive and honest way. I share their stories, fears, hopes and tears with the hope that this collective diary will provide comfort, assistance and a little light relief to you, my sisters and friends.

The Start of the Meno-madness

Human being to a raging goddess in sixty seconds

I wish I had known what menopause was before that trip to the supermarket in the summer of 2019. My dad always had a Jamaican saying which went "those who feel it know."

Well, I wish I knew then what I know now.

Let me start at the beginning and tell you how it all began...raging hormones, the warm weather and my lack of knowledge and awareness of my current affliction. Let's just begin with that and for the rest, I'll plead the fifth.

It was a sunny, Sunday afternoon and I was with my handsome son, my eldest child. As usual, my beautiful fifteen-year-old daughter was out playing her beloved football and had no interest in accompanying us for a trolley full of meat and vegetables. We decided to go to the local supermarket and as we approached the entrance, just off the main road, I glanced to my left and saw four teenagers messing around at the side of the road.

I notice teenagers. This is probably because I spent the first twenty years of my career working with underprivileged youth in various capacities. I loved my work and put years into supporting these young people to build their self-esteem. I would help them see that they could reach their full potential and achieve their dreams.

This was a natural extension of my childhood and I believe I could connect to young people easily due to my own 'colourful' past. I choose the word colourful carefully and still as a front. When you go through specific painful experiences, I believe you have a choice to let them make you or break you. These are the affirmations I learned to tell myself to bring out my inner strength, and it seemed to work. Painful childhoods never go away, but they can lift you in many ways if you learn to change the narrative. That was a lifetime ago and I now believe that kids are a different breed altogether. It's not their fault, but it is scary at times. I can only think that the total lack of respect that some kids have, comes from the demise of any kind of authority or discipline figures, but that is another story. We proceeded into the car park, found a space and started shopping.

After moseying up and down the aisles for twenty minutes I came across the same group of teenagers which I had seen earlier. I was on my own at that point. My son had bumped into someone and was having a catch-up. One of the girls from the group was mindlessly pushing a trolley into other shoppers, literally moving it into them and laughing. Without giving a second thought using my left hand, I held onto the trolley and asked her in no uncertain terms what she was doing, to which she replied, "None of your f#%king business".

Well! My menopause did not like that and thought it would introduce itself to her. At this point it hadn't introduced itself to me yet either. I proceeded to hold onto the trolley so she couldn't go anywhere, oblivious to anyone else except for myself and this demon of a child who stood helplessly before me.

Fast forward a few minutes later. The reason why I fast forward is that I don't remember it at all. Some call it the Red Mist! Does this sound familiar?

The young demon is attached to the end of my arm, with legs dangling in the air. I held her clothes by the scruff of the neck as she pleaded with me to let her down, trying to persuade me by saying, "I'm only 14!!". That was it! The next thing I remember was screaming at the top of my voice, saying, "I don't care how old you are, what do you think you are doing?" With a good scattering of choice expletives, I followed it with, "Fix up and stop messing around".

Then, as quickly as the situation had escalated from nought to sixty, it simmered back down. Obviously, the demon child needed some sort of discipline! At this point, I was confident that she had learned her lesson speedily and she proceeded to act according to some kind of social norm. Can I just reassure you that no one was injured in this transaction.

I can vaguely remember other shoppers saying comments like, "Good on you love, the little scuffers", "Someone needs to raise these kids nowadays" and "It's like they were dragged up" but I have a very blurry and sketchy recollection of the situation.

The truth is, I have a lot of compassion for children like this. I didn't let falling pregnant with my first child stop me from studying for a degree in youth work. I had a mission and that mission was to help children just like this child. They say hurt people hurt people, but I believe that your path can go one of two ways. Hurt people either hurt people, or they strive to heal. Due to my own childhood experiences and my knowledge of working to help children with challenging behaviour, I usually have so much love and compassion for this type of child. However, neither my patience nor my empathy seemed to be present on this day. What had changed?

Out of the corner of my eye, I saw two shop workers who possibly asked if I was okay. I said yes and remember informing them what had transpired and why I was assisting a fourteen-year-old to learn to fly. That was it! With much huffing and puffing, my son and I continued shopping and reflecting on what had happened, obviously including my justifications for stopping the appalling behaviour of the 'demon' child. I vaguely remember thinking, what if this child hits an elderly person or a small child with that trolley, they could do some real harm. I'm an empath, so I am very much led by my feelings. Later, my son informed me that the child had hit me and maybe that was why I had reacted in the way I did, but to be perfectly honest, I didn't feel anything.

My son was chatting away to someone at the start of the encounter (I think it was his brother's mum) but he was quickly enlisted to the drama.

More worryingly, was the fact that he also told me that as I held onto the trolley, the other three friends of this 'demon' child, one female and two males, had stepped forward as if they were going to hurt me. My son said he quickly stepped in front of them and told them to "step back." He also said, "To be fair, Mum, I wasn't worried. You looked like you had everything under control."

The truth is that I have never felt so out of control in all my life.

On reflection, the reason I share this absolutely embarrassing behaviour on my part is to highlight how, at the peak of my transition into perimenopause, my hormones were raging and so out of control. I behaved in a way that I definitely would not have before, at least, not since I was a teenager. Admittedly as a teenager this could have been me. But after all the work I had done around finding my life's purpose and becoming the best me, I was now faced with a situation. This made me feel as though I had never reached any spiritual enlightenment before and I felt as though I had been living a lie for the last thirty years.

It highlights the immense and frightening behaviours that our bodies can go through especially when we are unaware of the changes that have taken place and why they have happened.

Unbeknown to me that wasn't the first time my menopause had affected my life. On reflection and in the spirit of total disclosure, I believe I started experiencing my symptoms a long time before that incident. The incident I described was definitely the most bizarre and out of character, but there were some funny experiences too.

I remember clearly, returning from my honeymoon in 2016. My second husband and I got back to where we had parked the car. I had used a park and fly and as I waited for my car to be delivered, my husband and I chatted about our fabulous vacation. The car came back and I thanked the guy who dropped it off and we looked forward to the long drive back to my home town, or so I thought.

That's when the fun started; at least it's hilarious now, although I didn't think so at the time. I started the car and it was jerking back and forth. After several attempts to drive it, the poor engine finally died. I flipped! In my mind, as I remembered snippets of information and reviews that I had read online, where some customers had alleged that the company was driving the cars wildly while they had them. I went from nought to sixty, again, blaming the poor guy for driving my vehicle inappropriately and flooding my engine. I wouldn't stop. I was on a mission.

Someone had to be at fault, didn't they? After several minutes of ranting and Mr Car Park Guy looking bewildered with no apparent answers to my questions, I called the breakdown people. I was signed up to one at least, so that was one good thing under the circumstances. We waited for what seemed like forever, but was in fact only about thirty minutes, when an angel appeared disguised as a friendly breakdown man. I handed over the keys and the car miraculously started. Bless him, he took his time and drove it around the car park, doing a few other checks and then he admitted to not really knowing what was wrong. He assured me that if I drove sensibly, it would be fine. I was still nattering in the background, trying to convince him that the car park driver must have flooded my engine and that I was sorry it had appeared that I had wasted his time. Friendly Angel, disguised as a breakdown man, was most gentlemanly, said no problem at all and went on his way. He even waited until I had started the car and was heading out of the car park safely before he disappeared into the afternoon sunset.

Later, when I was driving down the motorway, I had a huge epiphany. I could see myself clearly starting the car a few hours earlier and I could feel my face begin to warm up as I realised that it was I who had flooded the car. I realised that I was driving an automatic car while on holiday, but my car was a manual. I could see myself trying to set off as if I was driving an automatic instead of a manual, hence the jerking back and forth. I felt so stupid. It was clear that I had forgotten to change my driving style. I felt like a horrible person for ranting at the poor car park man. To this day, I haven't used the car park in question again and I don't think I've ever told my second husband what happened. I'm not sure if he was unaware, being a non-driver himself, or kindly decided to ignore my foolishness so as not to make me feel any worse. Either way, I appreciate his approach.

Am I the only one who has suffered this affliction? Absolutely not. Although sometimes we listen to a story, which can make us smile or laugh, there can be a sad and dark side to menopause. It has been known to cause some difficult situations when women have been totally out of control and sometimes to a devastating conclusion. During my interviews, I have heard countless examples where women have experienced situations where they have felt "out of control" of their actions, experiences ranging from mild and manageable to terrifying and downright dangerous.

For these women, I want to make a stand and say that you are not alone. We all need to do better as a society to support you. I finally want to say, "Do not be afraid. Be still. Learn to breathe".

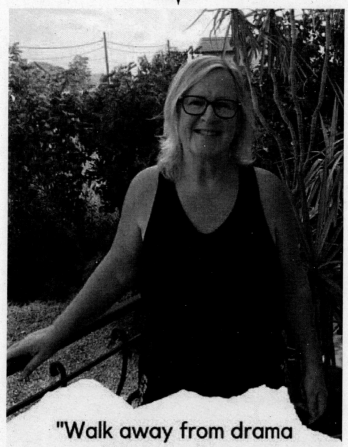

"Walk away from drama
and find time for you"

KAREN KEOHONE

Now let me introduce you to Karen K. Karen is an amazing lady who retired early from her long-standing job as a civil servant. She moved from her birthplace in Scotland and is presently living in Bulgaria, where she does whatever she wants. In Karen's own words, she says, "the choice to move to Bulgaria was to get away from the hustle and bustle of life."

At the time, she never really connected her new choices to her menopause but recalls that she only wanted a sense of freedom. She found this at the time, stating it was a form of self-preservation.

One day, Karen was having one of these scary experiences I just mentioned. Like most women will profess when experiencing similar things, the reaction was so out of character and so irrational. A response that she said was "way too much" for the actual situation.

I thank Karen for her bravery in sharing her story. I noticed something with most of my interviewees who had experienced menopausal symptoms that affect them emotionally. They seemed to have a certain embarrassment and sometimes self-loathing of their actions. They are blaming themselves first, feeling shame and guilt second and often continuing a berating dialogue with themselves for some time. In my opinion, it is unfortunate and some situations could be avoided or diminished with the proper care and support.

At sixty years young, Karen is in post-menopause and still experiencing symptoms. Karen discusses starting to have recognisable symptoms in her early forties. Karen continued in the perimenopausal stage for approximately ten years and wasn't even aware why she had started at the time either. Thinking it was because of pregnancy in her later years, having had her second and last child at age thirty-seven. Karen said that it never clicked at the time but she progressed to have raging hormones that were way out of control.

As a youngster, she only ever heard about menopause from her female relatives on the rarest of occasions and just as occasionally, in the hairdressers, where she was surprised that the clients were sometimes asked if they had experienced a hot flush. It could be felt on their heads during their pamper sessions, apparently. Karen said her dad and brothers would never have spoken about it, adding that her dad would have died if it had been mentioned. Karen playfully described the attitude and perception in Scotland based on her own experience: "This was a woman's crazy time, so stay away."

Even the women appeared not to really talk about it, but she did say, "They may have offered a little sympathy at times if you were going through a hot flush. Empathy would be shown, but that's where the communication and support ended."

Throughout her menopause, she endured at least sixteen identifiable symptoms but with no confirmation from anyone or anywhere that they were due to menopause. It is still a grey area for her to this day.

Karen tried only natural remedies in the form of herbal teas and a variety of capsules, which she feels helped her. They gave her a focus; something to think about other than her symptoms and particularly her irritability. She could focus on thinking about the remedy being tried and not about her behaviours or feelings. Confessing at times to being unaware, not realising it was menopause, she often felt as if she was going crazy. Sometimes ending up in floods of tears and heartbroken at the mere sight of an emotional advert, she would admit to having no idea why she became so emotional.

The scariest time was on a day trip with her partner and her children.

It all started as a nice day, driving along with her children in the back of the car. Then with no recollection of why, other than remembering her partner at the time rattling on and on about something, Karen pulled over the car and put her hands around her partner's throat. She proceeded to inform him that she was going to strangle him. Luckily, she did not! Eventually getting out of the car, she managed her actions herself by breathing and walking around. She describes the experience as a red fog or mist that came over her, with an uncontrollable feeling of being unable to stop. Karen describes it as feeling as if it was someone else and not her. Although she is aware that she did it, she was not in control of her actions. Karen said lots had happened around this time, but the main experiences were connected to rage and irrational behaviour.

Karen said that there were moments that could have been seen as funny or humorous, like when she wet herself whilst playing on her kid's trampoline. On reflection it seems most experiences were mainly scary for her.

Karen researched how to help herself, the main focus being her apparent anger issues. Feeling as though she was angry all the time at everything and everyone, Karen had a deep desire to understand what was causing that anger and what she could do to stop it. The irrational behaviour seemed to be linked to absolutely nothing that she could explain in any sort of justifiable way. Eventually, realising what it was and that this was not something that would last forever, life improved and Karen became calmer in the process. Karen was able to be kinder and reassure herself that she was going to be alright.

This awakening also prompted her to be fully transparent with her son and daughter. Karen has explained her actions to them now and discussed the hormonal links to her previous behaviours.

Apologies have been made and Karen says that her children have told her that she wasn't that bad. They reassured her that situations can feel a lot worse to the person going through it than to the people around you. Nonetheless, Karen still feels terrible, constantly questioning why she had to spoil the different events, such as a family meal or special occasions. With no advice, Karen had to work it all out on her own and feels that if she had been more prepared and aware of what was happening, she might have been more conscious of what she was doing. Karen's partner became her ex-partner; he didn't seem to understand her situation and what it was like to go through menopause. As most women often do, we make allowances for others instead of putting our own needs first.

Karen's ex-partner developed cancer, so he had his issues to deal with at the time. Sadly, he passed away, so she was never able to apologise to him directly. Karen, I am sure that he is looking down on you today, grateful that you finally found peace and for the fantastic job that you have done in raising the children.

When we know better, we do better.

Karen Keohone; our sister, our friend and our Queen.

Now, not all women experience a red mist, some women actually embrace their menopause. One such woman is Alicia who has been working as one of our faithful 999 emergency service operators for the past two years. She has previously worked as a foster carer and psychic. Like Karen, Alicia is fifty-two years young and originally from Dundee in Scotland. Now residing in Castleford, West Yorkshire, Alicia has been in postmenopause for approximately three years and started her first symptoms eighteen months before.

Unlike Karen, Alicia said that she immediately knew what was happening to her. Always expecting menopause around that time, Alicia got prepared from an early age. This was after hearing that women whose bodies had held many pregnancies had a higher chance of transitioning into menopause younger. Experiencing nine pregnancies in total, which sadly resulted in only three living children, Alicia also anticipated horrible symptoms like her own mother.

This may have propelled Alicia to be more prepared and put her armour on early. Luckily, Alicia doesn't feel like she had it half as bad as her mum.

Having never been given even one piece of menopause advice, Alicia had already done some independent research and welcomed the ending of her periods with open arms, although she had to adjust her mind to the fact that she would not be able to get pregnant again. Even though confessing to not wanting any more children, she admitted that she loved being pregnant, but this is something that has now been taken away and is out of her control. "It took some getting used to," she says.

In Alicia's experience, British people do not talk about menopause. She observed that the women she works with, who are experiencing this transition, are all very different. Not seeing it as an illness, personally, she thinks that it's something we will all have to go through as women, so we must learn to accept it. I think Alicia is our only sister who, during the writing of this book, confesses to loving the hot flushes...what a lucky lady!

Although exceptionally prepared and having a positive outlook from the start, she has still experienced seventeen recognisable symptoms. The biggest issue is the constant fatigue, when no matter how much sleep she gets, she still feels tired. Surprisingly, Alicia had an initial symptom that wasn't on my pre-prepared interview list. This was the development of a fetish for men in boots, especially men in uniform. It made me wonder if there was a link here with the recent career change to the emergency services.

Another positive thing recognised was a shift in her overall attitude. She basically feels that she doesn't care what others think anymore, instead choosing to dance to her own drumbeat: "I will speak my mind all the time and will always speak up for myself".

In the past, this wasn't always the case.

Seeing herself become emotional when she was never like that before, even at a sentimental social media video, has also been a transition to come to terms with.

Alicia confesses that the epiphany came when she noticed that she had finally had her last period. Realising that she was getting old, she made a conscious decision to live her life no matter what. It made her feel very aware of time and how little of it we may have left.

Not unaffected by those feelings of rage we have discussed earlier, Alicia confesses that little things like hearing people eat can still make her feel like murdering them, even alongside the positive outlook. Alicia feels that it's as bad as feeling like she could physically hit someone at times. Like others, she is aware that this feeling is totally out of proportion, saying honestly that her violent thoughts have increased one hundred percent. To date, these thoughts have not been acted out, which could be a good thing for those around her.

Alicia was prepared, so the changes seemed to be more manageable. It didn't stop her from feeling angry, nor did it prevent her from receiving two disciplinaries already in her new job for speaking her mind. However, she was able to control these feelings better. Was this why she was able to temper any outbursts?

There is a lot to be said for being prepared, allowing yourself time to adjust and prepare mentally. Thank you, Alicia, for taking the time to know yourself and find healing in the transition.

It was sad to hear that she felt someone had robbed her of her motherhood, a deep trauma for many, and we will delve deeper into this later.

I know it's not like this for every woman; in fact, I applaud those who don't have any effects on their emotions at all. But unfortunately, I'm not one of those lucky ones, so I just had to learn to breathe.

As I write these words to you, thankfully, I have not had any scary red mist episodes for at least a year and long may that continue and certainly, at the very least, for the sake of any young delinquents.

So, do all women rage? Of course not. Some can have a different kind of meltdown. One where you unknowingly become so sensitive that you can burst into tears watching mere adverts on the television, or so we were previously told.

Let's go find out what those days can be like.

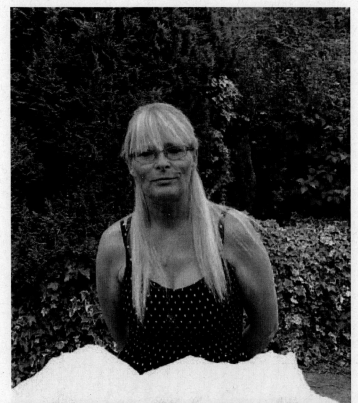

"Live your life better while you're younger. Don't just survive, but live"

ALICIA MULHOLLAND

From Rages to Babies

Does the madness ever end?

Growing up as a child who experiences trauma, you can learn that tears don't get you anywhere. I learned from a young age to put on my protective armour, or at least that's what you tell yourself. The armour sometimes resembled a hard shell, not caring about things or fierce independence. It wasn't true; I care deeply for many things but, when you feel so much pain as a child, you learn to protect yourself in any creative way that your mind will allow. But this learned behaviour kept me fulfilling what seemed like so much, when other people I knew seemed to struggle.

This was the fire inside me that propelled me to go off to college in the ancient city of York at just seventeen years old. I had chosen to study Art. The same fire helped me complete my studies, often on an empty stomach because I didn't always have any money for food. On one of those bad days, it was sometimes a packet of Super Noodles or a single package of Ovaltine from the corner shop, adding half of the recommended water as your mind tells you that a thicker blend will sit stronger in your empty stomach. I remember it well, twelve pennies a pack. It was the next best thing to having only a glass of water, which on rare occasions was sometimes all I had to get me through the long nights. My dad paid for my lodgings. If I told him that I wasn't eating, he would have made sure I was alright but I'm hard-headed. Since these were the arrangements we had made, I made sure that no one would see my initial failings.

I had a sister angel in the form of a lovely lady called Dawn. She was a lot older than me and she was kind, so I saw her as a mother figure. At the time, this was the energy that I craved, and the small child in me still does today. Dawn always looked after me.

After a while, she started bringing packed lunches for the two of us to eat our lunch together. I remember that Dawn was a single mum on benefits, trying to get herself through school. A few years later, I returned to York to pay Dawn back for all her support. Obviously, she laughed at me and said, "Don't be daft", but I always remember my angels. Angels who have guided me, supported me, and lifted me up at different points in my life. We all need angels, and we can all be angels to others.

The same passion encouraged me to learn to drive and buy my own car the same year, getting a job in a fish and chip shop so that I could get my dinner for free. I thought this was a clever idea at the time. It must have been because I don't remember being hungry after that. Realising that all I needed was some money to open up the possibilities I desired, I put my energy into getting as many part-time jobs as I could fit around my courses. I believe earning money became an addiction. It meant that I didn't need anyone, therefore nobody could let me down. I never thought about the issues this might cause my children later in life, if they never had me around.

Eventually, I moved back to my hometown. I soon realised that although I enjoyed Art, as it gave me peace, my logical mind told me it wouldn't give me a successful income.

Looking at my peers every day, I saw them as talented but myself as only okay. I didn't want to admit this at first, as Dad had already warned me of this before starting Art school. He never actually told me I couldn't make it but he asked me many times if I was sure that this was what I wanted with my life? I knew what he was implying. We sometimes do this to our children without realising it. We put our own past and limitations onto them under the guise of protecting them. It's limiting and can cause our children to move out of alignment with their own life purpose. Dad wasn't the first. I have been guilty of this myself and I'm sure many other parents have done this as well. With that, I decided to come back home and look for something more suited to my own skill set. At that time, I had no idea what this was.

One day, whilst attending a local college with a friend who was enrolling herself, I decided to register for a Health and Social Care course. This was mainly because I wasn't sure what to do, so I wanted to fill my days. Little did I know that this would spark my interest in helping people. Twenty-eight years later, I'm still in this field, currently the CEO of my own Homecare company.

Whilst on the course, I had three jobs. As a nanny, I arrived in the early morning to take the children to school, picking them back up at three. While these children were at their own schools, I worked as a teaching assistant in a local primary school as my second job. In the evenings, I worked as a youth worker. I don't know how I fitted it all in with my studies, but I did.

After this course, I went to the University of Leeds to study Youth Work. In the summer before I started, I discovered I was pregnant. Some people I cared about were disappointed and concerned because, after being a difficult child myself, I was finally getting serious about life.

They probably thought that having a baby at this point might take me back off track. I can understand why they would think that. That said, I love a challenge. I shifted gears and successfully completed my Diploma. I achieved it alongside working part-time, having my child, buying another new car and going abroad to do my work placement.

I remember people asking how I managed to do all that as they told me about their placements in the local shelters or schools. My answer was always the same. One foot in front of the other. It confuses me when I read articles about women being asked to move from restaurants because they are breastfeeding. I breastfed my son in the front row of my lectures until I got him into a nursery. I don't know if it's my aura, but nobody ever asked me to move.

Raising my children as a single parent, I gave them what I thought was a good life. I provided them with all the material things they wanted. We went on fantastic holidays, had a lovely home and a nice car. I didn't let things stop me from achieving what I thought my heart desired. This didn't come easily. I evolved over the years. I practised self-reflection and developed my self-esteem. But it's hard to erase a whole childhood of learned behaviours.

I think this was a particular issue in my first marriage, which barely lasted a year. My first husband was a chivalrous man, wanting to take care of me. At the time, I did not have that kind of strength. Allowing myself to be vulnerable was way too scary. I saw crying as an emotional weakness and emotional weakness was not a part of my plan. I devised mantras that ensured that I stayed '"strong"', choosing to tell myself I could do anything and nothing could stop me. The world was my oyster. So, I fought to stay self-sufficient. Ultimately, I had to let my husband go.

I don't recall exactly when the floodgates finally opened but it was some time between 2016 and 2020. I remember becoming a blubbering wreck. Whilst at work, in the middle of a meeting, discussing something completely neutral, my eyes would well up for no reason. I recall having to apologise to my colleagues and taking a moment to catch myself. I remember once sitting on the edge of my bed and crying inconsolably. On one occasion, my second husband, who may still have cared a little at the time, walked over, gave me a hug, and asked me what was wrong. All I could say from behind the tears was, "I don't know."

Because I didn't know. It's a strange feeling. Firstly, crying so much when you are not used to it, but even stranger was to be crying with absolutely no idea why.

I reflect back at this stage as one where I was very teary and totally not in control. I was becoming more emotional. I would cry at things I wouldn't have cried at before.

As I've said previously, I'm an empath. I am very used to being in tune with my emotions and those around me but I noticed it much more than before. If somebody started to talk about something and I recounted it in my head or something else reminded me of a situation, such as a sad image or a sad song, I could instantly become teary-eyed. I remember apologising on many occasions when my emotions took hold during work meetings. I would take a few minutes to catch myself and apologise for my lack of control.

That being said, not being overly stiff or unemotional previously, I thought I had learned that showing feelings were okay. I thought I had control of the overall base of my emotions, but this was a change that I was not prepared for in the slightest.

Starting to tear up in the middle of work meetings was very new to me. If I were to be totally transparent about my relationship with my emotions, I would say that I definitely felt everything before this. However, I was very controlled about sharing my emotions before this and it took a lot to cry in front of people. Usually, if I wanted to reflect on something emotional, I would do this in the solitary space of my bedroom with no audience and no judgement, but this was now a distant memory.

I don't think that I can recall the different scenarios of why I became emotional. Looking back, it seemed to be most of the time or at least once or twice a week. For the most part, there just wasn't a reason. A massive wave of emotions would just come over me. I know for many women, it is much more compounded and definitely affects their lives more intensely. Maybe because I was predominantly cursed with the rage affliction during my menopause, I did not pay too much attention to the tears.

There was one time that I can remember clearly. I had finished my garden project, and as I placed the last bag of bark down, with rake still in hand, my son stood by my side and I started to blubber. Not a little weep, I might add. This was a full-on, uncontrollable blubber. I felt every wave of emotion that day as I recounted the months of hard work that my aching body had endured. I cried for the project's beginning and end, the moments of fun, arguments, laughter, and tears in between. I cried for the progress my son and I had made, both in our relationship and as human beings. My son looked at me with concerned eyes and asked me what was wrong. After all these waves of emotions, all I could say, whilst I felt the magnitude of feelings was, "It's just so beautiful."

Aside from the angry menopausal rage and the other colossal emotions that some women go through, becoming overly sensitive and crying much more than usual is a real thing!

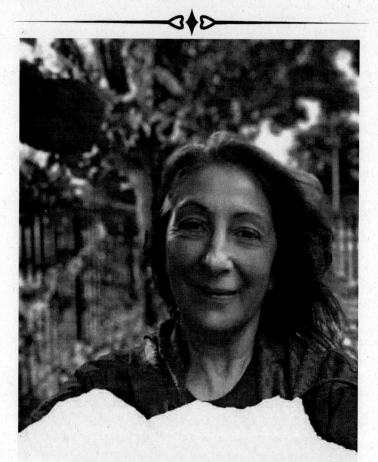

"Be kinder to yourself"

JO-ANN EISENBERG

Meet Jo, a sixty years young artist currently in post-menopause. Unaware that she was experiencing her perimenopause, she is now taking Hormone Replacement Therapy (HRT) and not wanting to come off it for fear of feeling the symptoms as profoundly again. Since starting HRT, her symptoms have basically stopped, with only the slightest minor signs creeping through on occasion. Born in Cheshire in the UK and now living in Leeds, she designs the most amazing stained-glass windows, teaches in community groups, and loves to spend time in her allotment.

The first time Jo ever thought about menopause was when she was asked by a lady in a health food shop if she thought she was in menopause. This was because Jo had gone on a mission to find something to help herself sleep. In her late forties, she confessed to not having thought about menopause before and was quite taken back by the suggestion. She felt she was far too young.

After this bold woman's suggestion, Jo found it hard to get this new idea out of her head. Already going through many personal challenges, she didn't link menopause to the other trials she was experiencing at the time.

Jo has experienced seventeen recognisable symptoms throughout her journey. A symptom that particularly resonates with Jo is that she has become very intolerant of people whom she does not want to be around.

Jo told me that she visited her GP so many times when her life seemed to be spiralling out of control. Even with the vast array of symptoms that she was experiencing, not once was menopause suggested.

Jo still endured the symptoms for eight years, though. Due to the scaremongering about HRT that she had heard, Jo was initially worried about taking it. Her GP explained that HRT has changed so much now from what it used to be. They explained the many benefits that it could have on her health. After trying many different natural products that didn't seem to do anything positive for her symptoms, Jo has now been taking HRT for seven years. Unable to handle the sleep deprivation any longer, she took the leap.

The decision to begin HRT was not one Jo took lightly, but since taking it she now is able to sleep.

Now aware that people did not talk about menopause before her transition, Jo admits that she knew absolutely nothing about the subject. It was never spoken about with her mum. Jo feels that her lack of conversation about menopause is more of a generational thing. The older generation does not want to talk about it and expects women to simply get on with it.

When Jo finally understood what the symptoms were about, she said she felt so happy that she felt like celebrating. This again confirms that women can feel much more empowered when they are aware of the changes they are going through. To Jo, it confirmed that there was nothing wrong with her, so she decided to embrace the negative stigma surrounding it. Jo feels she can now comfortably speak to friends in her own peer group. Since the revelation, she has instigated some exciting conversations about it with both men and women in her community Art classes.

How does Jo's experience fit in with this chapter? Jo experienced a real emotional rollercoaster before she started taking the HRT. At the time, in a problematic relationship, she encountered many emotional outbursts. Even mid burst, she would question her behaviour and tell herself that this was a weird situation.

Often getting very upset over things and overreacting, but unable to stop herself. Everyday situations that would have previously been only a minor irritation, had now become a huge irrational deal. Switching from feeling angry to feeling sad, Jo remembers feeling quite helpless at the time. She could not help herself or grasp the situation because she was unaware of what was going on and why.

Jo said that she felt as though she was sometimes 'going mental', switching from one extreme to the other. The whole time, she felt as though she was living in a constant state of anxiety and sadness, always with an underlying sense of impending doom. Even with people, Jo felt relatively isolated. She felt unable to connect with anyone, even people she knew.

Sadly, she felt unsafe most of the time. Her anxiety levels had elevated to disproportionate levels. Feeling so emotional, unprepared and not in control, she stopped going to social functions because of the constant isolation she felt. People then stopped inviting her because she was always saying no. This only further magnified the problem, it seemed like a constant, inescapable cycle.

Jo says that, to this day, her life has never returned to how it was. At first, she felt awful about it but has now finally adjusted her attitude. Although she still does not socialise much anymore, she is now okay with this new way of living.

Some readers, who have yet to embark on this journey, may feel as though all hope is lost. There is, however, some hope, as this is not the case for all. Even with the worst of symptoms, with the right kind of support and understanding, women can come out the other side stronger, wiser and freer.

Some do literally go through the whole process and barely even notice the change. One of these women is Ama who is fifty-six years young and living in London.

Ama is originally from Ghana and currently owns her own care company like me. She was a nurse in an Accident and Emergency department when she started her menopause. Ama is one of those people who tells me she barely noticed a thing as she transitioned.

Ama felt that she started pretty early, at fifty years old. Ama is post-menopausal at the time of writing but does not think she would identify which stages she transitioned through. There was nothing to gauge except for changes to her periods.

Ama was aware of some of the symptoms through talking to her colleagues at work, who she said spent their days fanning themselves through their tortuous tropical moments. In Ghana, before moving to England at the tender age of twenty-three, Ama's mum told her that she had entered menopause. Ama's mum did not have any symptoms that she was aware of. But, before you all pack your bags and head off to Ghana, I have it on good authority that it is not a geographical thing.

Seeing herself as one of the lucky ones because the symptoms weren't present; she credits this to a good diet and daily exercise. I am not sure if there is any evidence that this is the case as many women I spoke to were very health conscious but still suffered countless symptoms. Ama said she has noticed no changes except for her periods ending. She informed her GP but never had any tests because she did not feel the need.

Having had children early herself, she feels that she has a lot of empathy for women who may marry late. Ama says, "When menopause takes their womanhood before having a chance to bear children, this is sad."

Other than childbearing, Ama feels that there is nothing that would stop her life from continuing because of her menopause.

Ama admits to feeling a deep sadness about motherhood, but this is where her feelings ended. She doesn't allow herself to be emotional about the situation.

To you both, Jo and Ama, I say, "know thyself, be still and surrender".

Surrendering was a huge deal to me. It meant literally surrendering everything.

The woman I used to be, the woman I was and the woman I would become. I had made mistakes, particularly those that would see me acting out wildly from my newly imbalanced hormonal self. I had to truly surrender. This was not an easy process, but I got there in the end.

Stay with me, and I will tell you how I went from a blubbering raging bull to a well-balanced serene and angelic human being...almost! But surrender did not come at this point because I still did not know what was wrong. I had been in perimenopause for several years, unaware that my body was being taken over by a new life force.

So, what is perimenopause? Well, let's move on to the next chapter of the menopause sh*t show to find out.

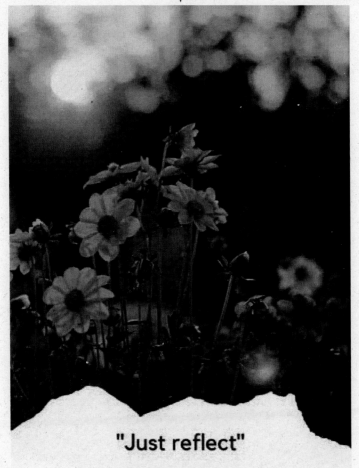

"Just reflect"

AMA OWUSUA

The Awakening of the Perilous Perimenopause

Medical GP or Doctor Google?

This chapter is for those who genuinely don't know what perimenopause is. It's where we explore the journey to finding out. It's the weeks, months and sometimes years leading up to menopause. It's where your body starts to experience the different hormonal changes. As I said earlier, I believe that I was in perimenopause for many years, though this was not even a part of my thought process at the time. Following my rage in the supermarket in 2019, I started to experience many different symptoms, which I did not link to anything remotely close to menopause. I think the reason for this was that in 2019 I was only forty-four years old. Much too young to even be thinking about it, or so I thought at the time.

In early 2019, I started to experience terrible headaches. Now I say terrible because I am not one to have headaches at all. In the first forty-four years of my life, I hardly had any headaches. So, in 2019 I got this monster of a headache. I usually have a glass of water and take a bit of paracetamol, but nothing seemed to help get rid of it. Months passed and it was becoming a real challenge. It was affecting my moods and I was staying in bed way too much. I decided to make an appointment with the doctor, who after examining me and asking general questions about my current life, was curious to see if I was suffering any known stress. Checking my records to find that many years earlier, I actually did suffer some stress headaches briefly. I explained that I was not currently going through any stress. The doctor responded with more information saying that stress can be present even if you are happy. I know that!! I'm the queen of stress, I was fully aware of this. Good stress, bad stress and the indifferent kind of stress.

I didn't believe that it was caused by stress because, by 2019, I was not working as hard as I had for the previous nine years when setting up my home care business. In those days, I would work seven days a week, fifteen to twenty hours a day covering all aspects of the company, from cleaning to care, payroll to accounts. Nowadays, life is actually pretty chilled, in my opinion. I had a great company structure and a fantastic team in place, which afforded me more time to breathe.

The doctor advised me to get some rest, plenty of water and relax, so I booked myself for several Thai massages...what better excuse? Then I tried to rest as much as I could. But it didn't end there. I progressed, starting to forget words, which was quite scary to say the least. Then my words would constantly get jumbled up whilst I was trying to form sentences. Now, this was definitely a negative experience. As a registered manager, I had a lot of responsibility, so my immediate thoughts went to what if this affects my obligations? What if I put any of my clients at risk by forgetting something important? After putting up with this experience for several months, remembering what the doctor said several months previously, I decided to go back.

Working with vulnerable adults, I was not a stranger to the symptoms of a stroke. I began to constantly check my face for any drooping because it seemed so unreal. How could somebody suffer from a headache for so long? At this point, my headaches had been with me constantly for about six months and by this point I had literally forgotten how to speak. Even wondering if I was developing dementia? Forgetfulness was the sign and I forgot everything. I was experiencing extreme tiredness some days, just staying in bed for no reason. Even watching my life pass me by would have been way too much effort.

I didn't want to try and hide it. I would find any excuse to curl up and climb into bed, only getting out for essential human functions.

The GP did some blood tests and I was low in quite a few vitamins and minerals. I say a few, but there were about four or five deficiencies. I definitely know it was iron and vitamin D, but I don't remember so much about the others.

The GP advised me to eat my greens and informed me that I had sticky blood. There was definitely a technical name when I consulted Doctor Google later, Antiphospholipid syndrome (APS), also known as Antiphospholipid Antibody Syndrome and Hughes Syndrome, but I definitely couldn't pronounce it. Going to Doctor Google later that evening, as we do, I was made aware that sticky blood was not a great thing to have but could also be caused by something as minor as an infection. I found out that it could also result in tiredness, forgetfulness and a person suffering from anxiety. This didn't help.

My doctor advised me that I should come back for more blood tests in four weeks because of the sticky blood. He was more concerned that I could not speak at times and that I had forgotten my words. So, the doctor made an appointment for me to go and talk to a consultant neurologist. Obviously worried, I anxiously awaited the meeting, which to my surprise, came through pretty quickly.

I told my husband at the time and although he didn't tell me what he thought, he attended the appointment with me. Because I was suffering from migraines, I went to speak to the specialist, head still pounding. The specialist was a lovely man and did a few random tests in his office. He said he wasn't perturbed, but he would like to send me downstairs to have an MRI just for peace of mind. He told me that the MRI screening would prioritise people coming from the emergency department first, then people who had actual appointments, so I may have to wait a while. I went downstairs for the MRI and waited probably about two hours. I then had to call the specialist asking him to send me an appointment in the post. The hospital lights and my headache were making my head feel like it would explode.

So, whilst I waited for the official MRI appointment, I started eating spinach every day, thrown into the blender to make a smoothie (see chapter 15 for some fantastic simple recipes). This was a first for me, but in fairness, they tasted beautiful. I blended the spinach with banana and strawberries or banana and mango. Sipping on them daily. I completed the course of iron tablets and a high dose of vitamin D, which was given to me by the original doctor. I generally made a conscious effort to eat more fruit and vegetables. Before this, I definitely did not have a high concentration of fruit and vegetables in my diet.

Then my appointment came through for the MRI, which I attended and I was seen swiftly. I got the results back within a week and the result was good news. There was absolutely nothing wrong with my brain, well according to the scan at least! But anyhow, I was at least put at ease once and for all. By now, the headaches had actually almost subsided and I had started to feel like myself again.

One week later and another trip to the original doctor to have my blood retaken, they were now happy that my vitamin content was showing as normal. I asked my GP if he had any idea why I forgot words. I said, "I'm still having trouble speaking and if there is nothing wrong with my brain, what do you think it could be?"

All he said was, "Who knows?"

I then asked if he was sure it couldn't be purely because of the vitamin deficiencies, because the symptoms had definitely improved since completing the prescription. My headache had finally disappeared after months of constant pain. The GP just looked at me but still no answer.

The final check was my sticky blood, which had apparently gone down significantly. The doctor said it was still there but, as it is easing, I shouldn't worry.

I think I failed to mention that at the first GP appointment, I had been with Doctor Google first. By now, I had noticed that my periods were fewer and far between, so I asked my GP if he thought I might be going into menopause, to which he replied, "Definitely not...you're way too young." This was around November 2019.

For the next couple of months, I continued to be conscious of my vitamin intake as I definitely did not want to experience those painful headaches again. I had grown a more profound empathy for people who regularly suffered from headaches and migraines. I didn't give menopause a second thought. I had identified that my periods were fewer and far between. Still, to curb my brain fog symptoms, as it's often known, I continued to be conscious of my daily fruit and vegetable intake.

So to recap, I had been experiencing irritability, extreme fatigue and emotional changes in periods of rage, anxiety and tearful episodes. I had also experienced forgetfulness and irregular periods but still no talk of entering perimenopause or menopause from my doctor.

I know I am not alone and this is a sad and frightful thing. Some say that menopause is a new age problem, meaning that the average lifespan for women was forty for many years.

Technically, most women wouldn't have even gone through it, or so some say. I say that may well have been the case, but we are not in that century anymore. How long does it take for society to act appropriately when they are aware of an important issue? From what I know now, it's way too long.

Fast forward only a few months to January 2020, where I was swiftly informed that I was indeed in menopause following another blood test review. This confirmed that I had been suffering the symptoms for the last several years as I'd started to think. The doctor refused to entertain such a thought at the time, which only delayed my peace of mind unnecessarily.

So how is the transition for most women? Well, I'm no expert, but I'm definitely a talker. I speak very openly with most people I meet, informally all the time and to share this collection of diaries, formally. To give you as broad an idea as possible, I have spoken with women from across the globe of different ages, shapes, colours and temperaments.

Does temperament dictate or influence the outcome of doctors and medical professionals? As you know I have already highlighted that I have no issue challenging anyone, but what of those women who are not as confident? One such woman is Charlie.

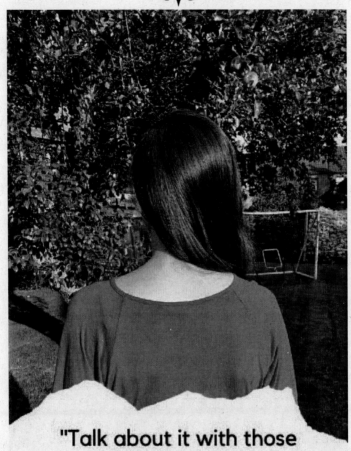

"Talk about it with those closest to you"

CHARLIE JENKINS

Charlie lives in Selby in the UK and works as a structural engineer. I don't think I told you earlier, but some of these amazing women I have known in different contexts and some are totally new members of my new menopause family.

Charlie is someone I have known for a while, not very long, probably about three years. I met Charlie as a football mum and we became football buddies. Charlie is easy to talk to, with a natural kindness to her nature. I could always rely on Charlie to save me a seat or grab a coffee for me if I forgot my purse (brain fog attends football games too). I remembered another funny thing I did when attending one of those football games held in another city. It was a sunny day as I watched our ladies play, sitting in my camping chair, chilling in the sunshine. I watched the game and our ladies won, which was the usual protocol. I might add that's an accurate account for the three seasons my daughter has been playing for her team, all fantastic players and the games are enjoyable to watch. The game ended, I came home and after driving forty minutes of the forty-five minute journey, I realised that I had come home, leaving both my handbag and camping chair at the side of the field. You can imagine what I was feeling, but thanks to a few thoughtful people from the losing team, I got all my items back in one piece. After their loss, I was so grateful that they were good sportsmen and didn't just leave it there.

Oh yes, back to Charlie, who always laughs heartily still when she remembers me leaving my chair as she also experiences her own periods of forgetfulness. As mentioned, there is also a sort of timidness to Charlie, which is hard to put your finger on, but if I was to wager a bet, it seems that Charlie lacks a little bit of confidence in herself. I find this hard to understand as ultimately, I'm the most confident person I know. When you speak to Charlie, she is so knowledgeable in so many areas, even her job as a structural engineer is complex, which makes it hard to acknowledge a justifiable reason why she would be like that.

She has the sort of aura that is love and light, mixed with a need for a hug, if that makes any sense? Let's put that aside for now and share her story.

Being fifty-two years young, Charlie feels that menopause has lasted a long time. Having experienced her symptoms for eight years, Charlie was in perimenopause for approximately seven years and has now been in postmenopause for a year. However, at the time of interviewing, Charlie wasn't able to clearly define what stage she was in, as is the case for so many women.

Sadly, Charlie equated many of her initial symptoms to possibly having panic attacks due to stress. Only when the night sweats became more profound did she start to recognise them as symptoms of menopause. It took a while and Charlie already had preconceived notions of being too young. Being in her forties,

Charlie said she wasn't expecting to see the 'big M' knocking at her door until she was in her fifties, at least.

Unlike many women, she did visit the doctors to talk about this new transition. The response she received was sad, with the doctor telling her, "It's not a disease, it happens to everyone. It's a natural thing."

Charlie felt as if the GP, who was a female herself, had "brushed her off."

As we speak, Charlie does that thing that women do. You know that thing we are all guilty of, where we make excuses for people and fail to put ourselves first? Receiving no guidance on what stage of menopause she was in, no guidance on where she could go for help, or where she could get any advice at all from anyone. It sucks! It's not really talked about at all by anyone, she recalls. "Where I'm from," she says, "It's an absolute taboo."

Taboo, baboo! As a child, I actually liked that word. It was a song I loved and a really lovely drink. But as I have approached my later years, it's become a word that I despise. For me, it represents asking us to shut up! And as I said earlier, that's just not my style.

Now Charlie was aware that menopause could affect your moods and she had preconceived ideas about HRT. Due to things that Charlie had heard, she felt that HRT was definitely a negative thing, but will admit now it was with no factual information at all. Isn't this where the doctor could have stepped in?

Experiencing sixteen identifiable symptoms, Charlie recounted behind her signatory nervous giggle as she admitted to experiencing an increase in irritability. She confirmed that she had allowed her emotions to take hold at times, snapping at those she loved. So again, it raises another question, that for someone who has some hesitation in life already due to her more insular personality, coupled with being a woman who often puts the needs of others first naturally, what does that do to you as a human being? As a woman? As a wife? As a mother? I doubt that this lack of care and compassion from the people who have taken an oath to do no harm has caused untold emotional damage to millions of women with this blasé attitude.

As with many women, admitting that the symptoms were the worst in the beginning stage. 'Horrendous' is the word that Charlie used to describe her night sweats, feeling low in mood at times and experiencing a feeling of letting sadness take over her. The effects of the sadness leave her with an aching dwell with no words to describe the reason.

A symptom not mentioned yet are heart palpitations, the scariest experience for Charlie. Unaware of what was happening and with a lack of knowledge, this frightened her a lot.

Feeling anxious about being anxious, Charlie worried if it would take hold so much that it would spill over into her job. She described it as a daily struggle to manage the anxiety that she experiences. With no real rational reason, it's just a dreaded fear that she will lose control of her feelings and responses.

Having one child, Charlie admits that there have been times where she has let her emotions take over her. I feel compelled to remind all these women that they are not alone. This appeared a challenging thing to share, but we thank Charlie for her honesty. One birthday, while having a small family party, Charlie remembers completely flipping and feeling a sense of rage taking over her. It was totally disproportionate. The resulting behaviour came in response to a comment that her daughter had made. It was such a minor thing, she says. Her response was awful and completely ruined the evening for no apparent reason. She said that trying to get yourself into a different mindset and out of the rage can be quite a difficult thing to do. The red mist meant that, in the moment, she was only able to focus on the comment and Charlie admits to beating herself up afterwards like many of us do.

I reassured Charlie that she was not alone.

An epiphany came when she realised that issues with the relationship between her and her daughter were not all her daughter's fault. She reflected on her behaviour and realised that she was an adult and needed to act that way. She would have to look at her input and learn to control what she said. She has spoken to her daughter and apologised with explanations about menopause and its effects. This is poignant because the timing of menopause can often coincide with our daughters' hormonal changes, which is why there can be fireworks.

The symptoms that our sister, Charlie, admits to being the absolute worst were night sweats and the resulting lack of sleep, which can do untold damage to our existence. Why should any of us have to suffer in this day and age? Why, oh why indeed.

Dear Charlie, today I would like to declare that I see your power. A beautiful soul shining bright in all its glory.

Lisa's experience was slightly more positive concerning the support she has received, which I am really pleased with. This may be due, in part, to Americans being more forward and not being backwards in asking for what they want. I'm not American, but I seem to have had more of a positive response from some doctors because I'm outspoken, so maybe there is something there.

Lisa is famously known as the owner of the Yummy Yank. Coming from Baltimore in the USA and now living in the UK, I first met Lisa when I still had my long-lived sugar addiction. I saw her selling the most amazing cakes at a food fair. I'm not sure if there are enough words to describe just how yummy they are and even though I don't eat so much sugar these days, I must admit that if I see her at a fair, I'm not sure I would be able to resist.

At sixty-four years young, Lisa is still reinventing herself and has a renewed sense of freedom.

Working through her symptoms, Lisa has been experiencing hot flushes for the last twenty-three years. Yes, twenty-three long years. The first signs came at forty-one with hot flushes arriving suddenly and her periods stopping. No warning, no initial signs, nothing. Believing that there was no perimenopausal stage, moving straight into full-blown menopause, the flushes that Lisa experienced were constant, day time, night time, and every moment in between.

Trying to be happy with the ending of her menstrual cycle was the thing that was difficult to come to terms with because she feels she started the transition so early.

Having a mother who, like most women, didn't talk about it, spurred Lisa on to talk lots and lots to her own children: "I wanted to seriously make sure that my kids can understand what could happen to them."

Lisa ponders her own daughter, who is now in her thirties with no child yet, hoping that her daughter can enjoy motherhood before it is taken away.

In the years that followed and after experiencing several different unrelated health issues whilst having a hysterectomy, the doctors found out that Lisa had Asherman's Syndrome. The doctor and Lisa discussed whether this condition, which she could have had her entire life but not known about, may have been the cause of the early onset of menopause.

During the hysterectomy, the ovaries were left, which sadly means that Lisa continued to endure all the hot flushes. However, most sweetly, Lisa confides that this is common practice for ovaries that are still healthy. Even though it has been a long twenty-three years she admits to coming to the realisation, she may have hot flushes for the rest of her life. Not experiencing a full night's sleep for twenty-three long years, Lisa giggles away and states that at this point, "sleep is overrated". What a woman!

Taking a little bit of time before approaching a GP to talk, Lisa says she was waiting first to see what happened.

The strength of women often amazes me as Lisa informs me that as a child, she went through some other trials due to a drug that her mum had taken while pregnant. The drug had adverse effects on some who took it, much like the thalidomide drug of the 1980s. From sixteen years old, Lisa was then signed up to years of testing and checks to ensure that the impact on her wasn't too detrimental.

Prior knowledge and awareness of menopause came not from any actual discussions with her mother but from merely watching her. Observing her mother in her 50s taking some sort of HRT, Lisa only became aware as a child visiting doctor's appointments with her mum. Remembering these times, she thinks this was due to several prescription changes to determine the correct dose. Not only didn't her mum discuss it, but neither did any of her aunts.

Having an older sister who started her menopause in her 50s, years after Lisa, there was no one in the immediate family to turn to. A blessing was a peer group of older ladies, who Lisa was at least able to confide in. Through discussions and some humour, they were able to support her through this initial transition.

Describing a friend, who had the sweetest nature, turn from "Dr Jekyll to Mr Hyde," Lisa knew that this menopause thing "was really something."

Sadly, Lisa likened the experience to having postpartum depression. She boldly states that, "it is a hormone exchange so powerful that if most women don't understand it, then how can we expect men to understand it either?" Lisa makes a valid point.

Lisa feels there is still a way to go in America's handling of the topic, although she thinks she has definitely observed positive changes in how it is spoken about over the years. People are much more open about it nowadays, with doctors giving you choices about what you would like to do. Lisa can see the difference between the two countries, in that she feels that in the UK, it is much more of a taboo subject.

Lisa had already stopped her regular checks concerning her mum's drug when she was pregnant, moving to the UK with her second husband. Lisa was convinced to resume regular testing again because doctors were fascinated about her condition and wanted to learn more. Not happy about this, mainly because the testing was uncomfortable, there was light at the end of the tunnel, and this meant that Lisa had a more positive experience of discussing menopause. Not with a regular GP, Lisa did have access to a gynaecological specialist and the talks were very open. Lisa giggles and says, "Well, I am American, so I make sure I talk about things. They had no choice really."

Although feeling that people laughed at her, she said she could speak about most intimate symptoms without shame, anything that came part and parcel with menopause. She was happy that she had access to an understanding doctor, who she adds has now sadly retired. Having been in the UK for twenty-four years, Lisa says she still can't get used to the feeling that GPs in the UK feel uncomfortable speaking about intimate subjects.

Lisa has experienced thirteen recognisable symptoms at different points of her journey and is still experiencing some to this day. The symptoms hit their peak around the fifty years mark and says they were non-stop for five years.

An added worry was that she had a sibling who developed early onset dementia, which led Lisa to feel overly emotional when she forgot something that her family might have told her. She says, "It's a strange feeling not to remember something that you probably should have."

Coming to terms with being unable to have another child was a scary realisation. Lisa says it is irrelevant whether she would have had another child or not, but it was a frightening realisation that this choice had now been taken away. Hard to come to terms with, probably because of the young age and losing the feeling of femininity and womanhood.

Listening to Lisa, she has such a sweet nature and positive outlook. It's breath-taking, considering the years she has endured these afflictions. With her support system of lifelong friends being four thousand miles away back in the United States, she is still finding funny moments amongst the challenges. Lisa laughs as she demonstrates how wide she flaps her tops when the hot flushes arrive, saying no matter where she is, "this is what I look like". Recounting a trip to Valencia where the restaurant manager, without a word, brought her a fan after she turned bright red while having a meal.

On a positive note, as I am privileged to share more and more women's stories. It is clear that a small number of women receive a good amount of support to help with their transition, but is it enough? Definitely not!

Are enough women offered the right amount of support? Absolutely not! But at least we can confidently say that it seems to be moving in the right direction for some women. I told Lisa that maybe she got a more positive outcome because she spoke to a specialist instead of a mainstream GP, which she wholeheartedly agreed was probably the case. Admitting that mainstream GPs just weren't equipped to handle dealing with the issue.

You might think I am labouring home the point about our sisters' lack of support and compassion. We are three chapters in and have only touched on a few of the plethora of different symptoms women can endure. If I haven't scared you too much up until now, let's talk weight gain and more pain.

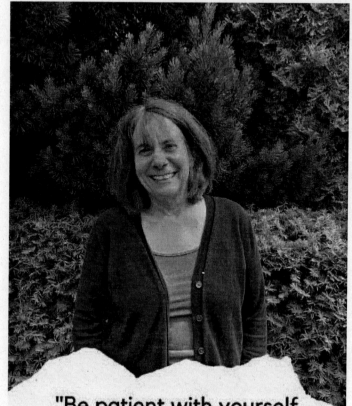

"Be patient with yourself and embrace who you are becoming"

LISA GAIR

Weight Gain...

And more pain

I'm not sure if I started at the beginning with this lovely affliction, but as I said before, I don't even know if I remember clearly when the beginning was? I know for sure that between 2016 and 2019 I went from being a size twelve to a size twenty; an increase of four full dress sizes! I got to the point where my midriff and stomach were so full of fat, I felt as if they were restricting my breathing.

It was uncomfortable to say the least, but as I will contest throughout most of my story, I was totally unaware and unable to connect the dots at the time.

It was definitely something I thought about when my children spoke to me, but not something I had thought of before; cue the lecture from the children shortly.

Now weight can affect many things; your thinking, your physical ability to do things and your emotions. This can include impacting your social life, when you find yourself making excuses for not going places because either you haven't got anything to wear, or you simply feel uncomfortable about attending whatever event you were meant to be at.

I think that the physical issues are the worst. Simple things like tying your shoelaces or walking up a flight of stairs become difficult and cause you to get out of breath quickly, maybe not in the beginning, but certainly over time. With most weight gain, it creeps up on you slowly, and because of this and the insurmountable changes that I was already going through, it took a while to notice the rut. I was sinking deeper and deeper into it. Let's call it a mindless state.

Then it's a downward spiral, isn't it? Cancelling appointments, comfort eating because you feel so bad about feeling so bad. However, I'll be honest, with all the other things still going on around me, weight management was at the back of my mind.

What I eventually did was start moving. I noticed that there was some healing to do in the relationship between my son and I. With this in mind, at the start of 2020, after my menopause revelation, I asked my son if he would help me do the garden. Little did he know that I didn't just mean cut the grass and pull out a few weeds. I'd been thinking for a while that I wanted a safe place, a haven...somewhere I could go to sit and meditate that was close to nature. I had a few things in mind and I will be honest the design unfolded quite organically and ended up a much bigger project than I had imagined. I started first by speaking to a friend of mine who is a garden landscaper. I explained that I wanted to do something beautiful yet simple and easy to manage. He gave me a couple of ideas, and I rolled with them. Initially, these ideas were to put down some garden mesh and make a few areas into different sections with bark and stones.

As I said, what manifested was something completely more exclusive and extravagant.

Six months later, my son and I were still toiling away. By the end, we had transformed the back garden, front garden and the side of the house. We got a pergola built with a roof, water features and flowers. It was our own little paradise. The overall theme was very zen-like. Anyone who had the privilege of coming to visit during the lockdown of 2020 was absolutely blown away, particularly for those who had seen it before. It has been a back garden which was just grass with a whole section of the back cut off and overrun with the dreaded ivy.

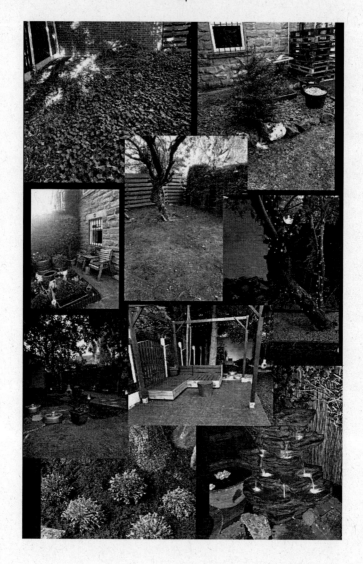

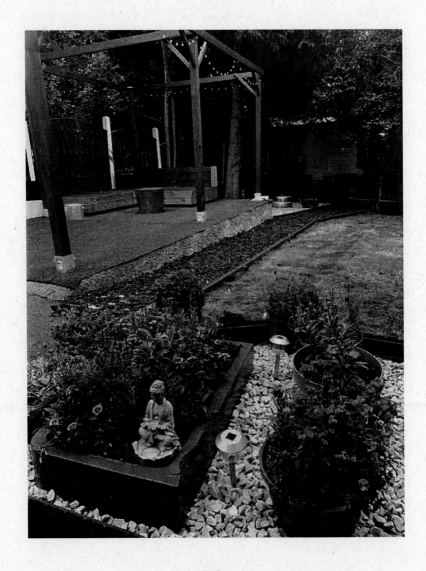

After a few weeks of moving my body, I realised that the aches and pains were starting to disappear, and I was naturally losing some weight. I had finally made the link between moving and feeling better, so I was eager to do as much as possible in the garden, much to my son's dismay. I remember having a couple of moments where I questioned myself, asking why I had started such an enormous undertaking? Clearly, it was because of my fierce competitive nature. I refused to be beaten, not by any plant, stone or piece of bark in any case.

I never saw myself as someone who had green fingers, but I always loved to be surrounded by nature, particularly water and any type of greenery. I would definitely advise anyone to make sure that they spend time in natural environments during this transition, either making use of your own garden, visiting local parks or nature reserves. I also let the garden spill over into my house and bought new plants to place inside. It helps to meditate around nature and helps me feel more grounded.

Weight becomes an issue for a lot of women during this time. It is not because we have done anything wrong or different, but because our bodies have changed. They need us to adapt to them. I found people not being compassionate around this subject and not understanding how menopause can work; for example, during a conversation with my son, he once said, "Mum, just start exercising harder."

He was unaware of the extreme amount of pain my joints were in, or the fact that I had learned recently that the body needs more relaxing exercises during menopause to combat stress. Our bodies are gaining weight due to hormonal imbalance. When I tried to explain this, he became unsympathetic and understandably so, because that's what we are taught for most of our lives. We are told that if we exercise harder, we will burn more calories. Granted, he did come back after doing his research and apologised. Due to the fluctuation and imbalance of hormones during menopause, weight gain is a common symptom. Exercises such as yoga and meditation can therefore be beneficial to reducing stress.

So that's a touch on the weight, but what other goodies have we got in store? Well, remember the chapter title: Weight Gain...and More Pain!!

There are so many different symptoms that women can go through, and we have only touched on a few of them. So, before we go any further, please read through the following symptoms so we can all get on the same page. If you don't get too scared, I'll see you on the other side.

Possible Symptoms during perimenopause, menopause and postmenopause

· Hot flushes

Periods when your body can heat up unexpectedly. Some women say that they feel hot around the head area, whilst others describe it as a heat that starts at their feet and rises all the way to their head. This is usually caused by the imbalance of hormones affecting your body's ability to control your temperature.

· Brain fog/ memory loss

Periods of forgetfulness, often described as brain fog. That feeling of going into a room and forgetting why you are there. Many women experience frustration as they forget words or how to string a sentence together. Short term memory loss or memory lapses are also common menopause symptoms. Part of this can be explained by sleep deprivation. Fatigue and other symptoms combined with hormone changes can cause you to become more forgetful. Usually, these memory lapses are temporary, and you can eventually remember what you were trying to recall.

· Weight gain

Women can gain weight due to fluctuating hormone levels and often gain weight around the abdominal area. Contributors to weight gain at menopause include declining oestrogen levels, age-related loss of muscle tissue and lifestyle factors such as diet and lack of exercise.

· Night sweats

Hot flashes that appear at night. Often causing regular bedding changes, insomnia and hot sticky feelings. Like hot flushes, this is usually caused by the imbalance of hormones affecting your body's ability to control your temperature.

· Difficulty sleeping

Being unable to sleep either at all or only being able to sleep for a couple of hours. This is usually due to night sweats but can also be due to low mood.

· Headaches

Experiencing throbbing, constant, sharp or dull pain in your head or face. Headaches during menopause are most frequent in adults who frequently had headaches accompanying their periods. When you get headaches due to hormone changes in the body, they can be challenging to treat.

· Low mood or anxiety

Anxiety can present as a feeling of impending doom for little or no cause. In extreme cases, it can lead to panic attacks which can be debilitating and painful. Some women feel mild anxiety simply due to the other symptoms they are experiencing and the fact that they are getting older. The fluctuation of progesterone and oestrogen can cause feelings of depression and anxiety. Serotonin and dopamine are affected by reduced oestrogen levels, and these mood-stabilising neurotransmitters can be responsible for high stress.

· Changes in libido

Changes in a woman's body and sexual drive due to the loss of oestrogen and testosterone following menopause. Menopausal and postmenopausal women may notice that they're not as easily aroused and may be less sensitive to touching and stroking which can lead to less interest in sex.

· Vaginal dryness

Vaginal tissues become thinner and more easily irritated resulting from the natural decline in your body's oestrogen levels during menopause.

· Sore breasts

Breasts being tender or sore to touch caused by the spikes in hormone levels affecting breast tissue. Breast soreness should improve once your periods stop, and your body no longer produces oestrogen.

· Irregular periods

Menopause is the transition into no longer having periods or producing eggs. Whilst in perimenopause, the length of time between periods may be longer or shorter, your flow may be light to heavy, and you may skip some periods as ovulation becomes more unpredictable.

· Joint pain

Pain that affects the knees, shoulders, neck, elbows, or hands. Because oestrogen helps to reduce inflammation, old joint injuries may begin to ache. As time goes on, you may start to notice that you feel more aches and pains in those areas than you used.

· Electric shocks

The feeling of light electric shocks can sometimes occur during menopause, usually lasting just a brief moment but can be pretty unpleasant. It is believed that this is due to the lower oestrogen levels wreaking havoc on the nervous system. It may feel something like a static shock and can occur anywhere on the body. Many people report that they get electric shocks across the forehead just before a hot flash.

· Dry tongue

Dryness of the mouth or tongue. Salivary flow rates are influenced by oestrogen levels and women in menopause have lower flow rates of saliva than menstruating women.

· Gum problems (metal taste in the mouth)

Gingivitis and bleeding gums are common among menopausal women. While this could result from ageing or poor dental hygiene, some studies have linked it to lowered oestrogen production which is what can cause gum problems during menopause.

· Digestive issues like flatulence and bloating

Experiencing bloating, increased gas, cramping, or nausea. This can be caused by changes in oestrogen levels and can disrupt the natural transit of food in the stomach and intestines, leading to some digestive issues. Bloating usually presents as fullness in the belly that can sometimes be painful and cause increases in the passing of wind. Bloating can occur during menopause as a side effect of digestive issues when hormone changes cause fluctuations in how food digests. It could also be related to irregular periods or hormone changes in general.

· Dry, itchy skin

Itchy skin that feels as though something is crawling on you is another symptom of menopause. The lower oestrogen levels in your body also lower the collagen in your skin. This can lead to thinner and dryer skin, which can cause an itchy or crawling feeling.

· Dizziness

Getting a spinning sensation, feeling lightheaded, and/or losing your balance. This can occur as a result of lowered oestrogen.

· **Fatigue**

feeling drained, overtired and lacking energy and motivation. Caused by dramatic fluctuation of hormone levels which causes the brain to wake up at all hours of the night. Also, lower levels of progesterone make some women short-tempered and less able to relax.

· **Loss of hair or hair thinning.**

Having hair fall out in noticeable chunks or noticeable thinning of hair but it may not always be as immediately noticeable. It may occur slowly over time and not be observable until the significant loss has already happened. Some researchers speculate that hair loss and thinning is simply coincidental and common among older women in general rather than being specifically a menopausal symptom.

· **Brittle nails**

Nails that split, peel, or are simply weak. Low oestrogen levels can lead to dehydration, which may cause brittle nails.

· Tight muscles

Muscle tension, particularly in the neck and shoulders. Lowered oestrogen levels result in increased cortisol production. Cortisol is also sometimes called the stress hormone. Increased cortisol can lead to muscle tension, particularly in the neck and shoulders, but can also occur anywhere in the body.

· Incontinence

Stress incontinence occurs when the bladder leaks when laughing or coughing. Urge incontinence is where the bladder gives almost no warning of being full and cannot be held despite your best efforts. And finally overflow incontinence, when the bladder empties without giving the signal that it is full. You may experience one or all three of these types of incontinence when you go through menopause, however, it is unclear whether this is a symptom of menopause or simply coincidental that many adults have incontinence during this age range.

· Changes in body odour

Having a noticeably different body odour. The hormone changes your body goes through during menopause can cause you to sweat much more profusely than you ever have before. Also, the changes in hormones themselves can cause changes in body odour.

· Irritability

The feeling of severe agitation, finding yourself less tolerant and more easily annoyed at things that did not bother you before. This is usually caused by the change in hormones.

· Allergies

The 'sudden' development of allergies. Imbalances of certain hormones caused by menopause such as histamine, cortisol, and thyroid hormones can result in allergy symptoms.

· Heart palpitations

Where you feel your heart beating faster than usual. This is usually caused by the drop in oestrogen.

· Osteoporosis

Weakening of bones, making them fragile and more likely to break. During menopause, oestrogen, a hormone that protects bones, decreases sharply. This can cause bone loss, which can lead to women developing osteoporosis during menopause because women have thinner bones than men.

· Difficulty Concentrating

Lack of concentration such as difficulty focusing on complex tasks. Multi-tasking may become completely impossible and you may also have trouble remaining engaged in reading or watching movies or television. This is caused by changes in hormone levels.

Please be aware that whilst these are all common symptoms of menopause it is always important that you seek medical advice.

So those are some of the main symptoms women might experience during their menopause. Let's take a breath and move on.

Now I hope that at the bare minimum, you now know that women who go through menopause may or may not go through the entire range of symptoms. I never wanted this book to be scientific, quoting medical references and other technical blurbs. However, I do think it's important to discuss the basics briefly as all the women I interviewed had some shocking revelations when presented with the number of symptoms I have highlighted.

Many were experiencing at least one, but most experience more. Often unaware that they were related to menopause, most said they just thought they were getting old and got on with it. I have always wanted this book to be an easy read. Something that anybody can pick up, read and apply, or go out and learn more about the science behind this. There are so many different symptoms that we can experience as women, and not surprisingly, many women were unaware that some were even associated with menopause.

We already know that we are all individuals. Some women experience more symptoms than others and at different intensity levels. Some women experience nothing at all. I have experienced twenty various symptoms up to this point. However, after speaking to some of our ladies, I feel pretty blessed. Although there were so many for me and some could be very intense, they ended pretty quickly. This is unlike many women whom I spoke with, who have had to endure them for years. There is no guarantee that they won't come back and come back more vicious, because this can happen. At this point all I say to myself is, fingers crossed, I think I'm over the worst of it.

One lady who thought she was over the worst was Karen M, a fantastic care manager from Leeds in the UK. Karen is fifty-eight years young and at the time of her perimenopause, Karen worked in customer services.

Starting perimenopause in her early 30s, Karen is one of those unfortunate people who, years after her symptoms ended, experienced a random "phantom" menopause about four years ago. Years after her symptoms had already finished, Karen, like many others, wasn't aware that there were different stages to menopause. Having a hysterectomy at thirty-one years old, she was told of the possibilities of going into early menopause. Karen immediately entered menopause and encountered symptoms for approximately four years. Symptoms were worse in the beginning and gradually eased off over time. Being given HRT patches to ease the symptoms, she was informed that there was nothing else they could do at the time. The patches didn't seem to help and Karen seemed to only gain weight. Feeling frustrated with the weight gain, she decided to stop.

Experiencing sixteen identifiable symptoms back then, she was only aware that menopause meant ending the menstrual cycle and experiencing hot sweats now and again. Hence why Karen wasn't ready for the array of symptoms that were to follow.

Karen recalls her mum being institutionalised for a short time due to her mental health becoming so bad that she was suicidal. Reflecting on it now, Karen wonders whether this had been a one-off incident whilst her mum was going through menopause. Back then, Karen wished it could have been dealt with better but there was a real lack of support and information available to women at the time. Karen also commented on the British way of keeping a "stiff upper lip", a far cry from the more open dialogue and experiences in the US.

Karen recalls a terrifying episode of her own. Following a period of not sleeping well, Karen returned home from working all day to look after her kids. She managed to fall asleep for a little while. Karen awoke later that night, convinced someone was trying to hurt her. She managed to call her mum, telling her "They're going to get me!"

Suffering from sleep deprivation, Karen had ultimately gone to sleep and woken up in a nightmare. Only being offered a psychiatrist in the hospital, she feels the medical response was less than helpful. Karen doesn't remember associating the symptoms with menopause, even though the sleep deprivation went on for some time. It was the scariest feeling that she had ever experienced. Following this, she only dared to finally get some sleep when her mum promised to sit and watch her. Sleep deprivation is no joke and the possible effects should not be underestimated.

Constantly feeling teary with heightened emotions, Karen explains the feelings as not rational.

She could recount a few fun times, one of which she remembers leaving her son outside the butchers. Shopping with her mum in Leeds, her mum went to buy eggs, leaving Karen with one child in his wheelchair. Karen can laugh now as she recounts meeting back with her mum, who promptly asked where her other son was and realised that she had left him outside the butchers. I will never again feel guilty for leaving my chair and bag on that football field. Brain fog is a real thing. At least Karen saw the funny side and swiftly went back to get him with no harm done.

It took a long time for Karen to reflect back and make the links between all the emotions she was feeling and menopause. Being told by parents whilst growing up to just get on with things, her mum said it's part of the cycle of being female. Karen continued to perform her duties as a single parent, ignoring her own needs during this challenging time.

Well done to another Queen for making it through the other side, and we're sorry that you had to go through this. Unaware, unsupported and unguided, you made it and did it with style, raising your two beautiful children and then adopting two more. You should be proud of what you have achieved. Let's hope that the stories we share will go some way towards helping the next generation of women through this transition.

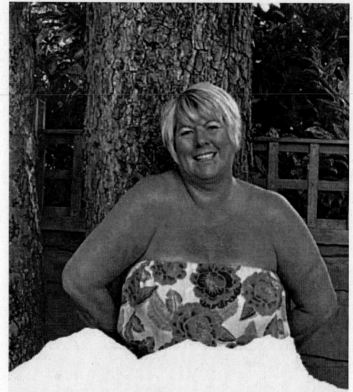

"Research and take time for yourself"

KAREN MILLER

Another lady who had an experience of symptoms that came right out of the blue was Mastaneh. At the time this put her in a dangerous situation.

Mastaneh, a fifty-six years young lady from Iran now living in the UK, is also one of my beloved football mums. Mastaneh has always worked and is not sure what stage of menopause she is in. The reason being is that Mastaneh has historically suffered from cumbersome and painful menstrual cycles.

Having two children close together, she was given the coil to support her with this. Periods stopping can also be a symptom experienced when you use the coil. So, although experiencing the symptoms, Mastaneh has never had it confirmed if she has gone into menopause. Not wanting to come off the coil for fear of re-living the destructive menstrual cycles, she has felt free for the last 17 years, as she doesn't get any stress now her periods have stopped.

Mastaneh informs me that the Iranian term for menopause is Yaissigi. Hearing about it from her aunts in Iran at a young age, she recounts their explanations of hot flushes. In Iran, far from being taboo, Mastaneh says it's normal to talk about menopause; at least for women, anyway.

Mastaneh told me about her symptoms. At times, she was asked by her mum to get something from the pantry and forgot why she was there. Mastaneh laughs as she recounts her mum joking with her, saying that she doesn't seem like the class A student of days gone by. One day, on a serious note, a terrifying situation occurred. Mastaneh experienced a blackout. She had dropped her daughter off at football training along a road that she had travelled many times before. On her way back home, she was alone. Whilst driving along, Mastaneh became lost. All of a sudden, she didn't recognise where she was. Slowing the car down, not only did her surroundings suddenly become unfamiliar, but she also had no recollection of where she was going. This went on for a few minutes, and really panicked her, before it finally clicked in, and she started to recognise her surroundings again. Does any of this sound familiar? I'm no doctor but it appears that Mastaneh was suffering from the dreaded brain fog. Guess where Mastaneh got sent next? Yep, that's right, a neuro specialist. Nothing was found. As we speak, Mastaneh is awaiting her MRI results.

Never having spoken to her husband or children, she admits that others have mentioned menopause to her several times. When observing her symptoms, people have asked if she is aware that her symptoms could be menopause. Mastaneh just laughs and admits she doesn't really want to know. With her fingers crossed that her forgetfulness is nothing more serious, the thought of painful and inconvenient periods keeps Mastaneh from finding out.

Mastaneh, the Sisterhood wishes you the best of luck.

So why do our bodies decide to put us through all of this? Well, I can only talk from my own experience, as I have briefly said already. When I started to look after myself better, eat better food, and do gentle exercise, I felt much better. Meditation helped a lot, lowering any external stress.

Obviously, this is a book, so I didn't want to give it all away in one go. What's next, you might ask? Can there really be any more? I'm sorry to tell you, but of course there is. I decided to give the next topic its own chapter because it seems to be such a sensitive one. This thing has been referred to as a symbol of women's femininity, their crowning glory. For years, women have been able to play different roles by changing different styles. From their stories, we can see that this contributes significantly to a woman's self-esteem. Yes, that's right! Let's talk about 'hair'.

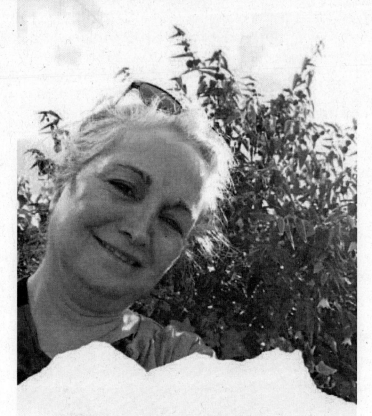

"Share your experiences"

MASTANEH AZIZI BABANY

Hair Today but Gone Tomorrow?

I am my Sister's keeper!

When I realised that the fear of hair loss was 'an actual thing', I must admit my first thought was that I had never been that bothered about my hair. For years I have just scooped it up in a bobble and got on with whatever it was I needed to do. I decided to spend a whole afternoon thinking about the relationship my hair and I had before even attempting to write anything of value for my sisters. I knew that I had to ensure that this chapter gave it the reverence and attention it deserved. Six days, five bouts of laughter and four inconsolable crying episodes and I finally reached some understanding!

Although I may not have consciously thought about it before, on reflection I learned there were deep seated traumas that this hair journey revealed. Firstly, it reminded me that for many women, their hair is their crown of glory. Secondly, although I thought it wasn't for me, it really was! It was just not at the forefront of my mind.

When I noticed that my hair was falling out, I was sitting in the salon chair. My hair specialist asked me if I'd noticed it was coming out in clumps. Now to be fair, I had seen that my brush was much fuller, but when she showed me the back of my hair with a mirror, oh my goodness, what a shock! It was all different lengths. I honestly had not noticed until she pointed it out. When she did, I must admit, I didn't feel scared. I felt fully protected by her knowledge and skills. Even though I had noticed the brush, I didn't make the link between the hair loss and my menopause. This doesn't seem unusual because after interviewing so many graceful queens, it seems commonplace for women to experience this sudden loss of hair. Immediately she recommended I give my hair a cut and treatment to get it all the same length and bring back the fullness. I made an appointment to come back in a few weeks, and she chopped off at least five or six inches, if not more.

As I looked at the new hair rug on her shop floor, I remember thinking the last time I cut my hair this much was around ten years before. I remembered getting a dramatic cut following a breakup. Women seem to do this, don't we? This amazing lady worked her magic, chopping and styling until I had a beautiful new bob, bringing back the fullness and overall quality. Looking at me and reminding me what I should be doing to keep it in the lavish style she had created. I could see the conversation behind her eyes as she confirmed to herself what she knew already. I wouldn't follow her advice. Not that I didn't respect her advice. It just wasn't me.

Deep in thought, I wondered where I had learned that my hair wasn't an important part of me. Over the years, I encountered a few hair horror stories, one of which I remember was sitting at a bus stop on the way to school. I used to always wet my hair in the morning to try to tame it. Having this 'wild, unruly afro', I was never taught to look after it properly. I wasn't given any hair products, and I certainly didn't have any assistance in making it beautiful. I had to work it out for myself. I remember sitting there playing with my hair and feeling these blobs, taking me a while to realise that it was the water that had frozen on this cold winter morning. I lived far from the bus stop, so I just had to try to warm it up with my fingers. I remember running into the bathroom as I arrived at school, anxious to fix the problem before class. Obviously, the only thing I could think to have done at the time was put my head in the sink and run some warm water over it again.

My dad used to work nights and one day when my favourite uncle, Evan, was looking after me, he put my hair into a braid. This was the first time my hair had seen any black culture at all and I remember really loving my new style. Unfortunately, the next time I saw these awesome braids being done was with another family who also used to look after us. Braiding all the kids' hair for school in the garden, one at a time, all the female children lined up. I watched as they all screamed as the adults yanked their hair with a fine-tooth comb trying to get the knots out. This put me off. I was about seven or eight and subsequently, my hair didn't see another braid until I was twenty-one.

Between the ages of nine and twelve, I lived with my mum. These are the years when I was finding myself and learning my identity. They were also the years when I endured most of my childhood trauma. My mum had her own needs and these didn't include putting her children high up on her list of priorities. I remember wearing make up every day. In fact, I wouldn't leave the house without it. I also spent many hours locked in the bathroom, putting conditioner in my hair. I had worked out that it made my hair a bit softer. Learning to comb my hair when smooth, I remember realising that not only was it softer, but it also hung down with the weight of the conditioner so I could mimic the flow of European hair. This meant that I tried to keep it on for as long as I could.

When I was about thirteen or fourteen, I started a craze between some of my friends. I decided to shave my hair at the sides and dye it like a chessboard. Those who have experience with afro hair will know that it does not 'just go blonde' with a packet of hair dye. This was my original plan, but I ended up with this obscure copper colour instead. That didn't stop people in my inner circle from following my lead. Our whole posse. Yes, that's right, I was in a posse. The fire posse. I remember it well. They all decided to follow suit, except for one friend. She refused to follow our lead and used common sense instead. I really don't remember what experience I had that led me to think it was cool, but I must have seen it in some movie or something.

I had a friend at the time, who had hair shavers and I just went for it. Short at both sides and longer down the middle. I know I still have some photographic evidence somewhere hidden in the depths of my attic.

One day, the last member of our crew asked me to do hers too. A willing participant, so I told her I would oblige. Without giving it any thought and not registering that the friend with the hair shavers wasn't present, I got to work with a Bic in hand. It didn't take long for me to realise that a Bic razor was not a clever tool to use for this job. As I observed the bald patch at the side of my friend's hair, my other friend (with common sense) and I looked at each other and started to laugh. Luckily our friend saw some humour in it, her mum however, gave us a right telling off. Looking back, I remember the same friend taking a few days off school to allow it time to grow.

The last story I want to mention at this point is that of my cousin. You will understand why when we get to the end of the chapter. My cousin Sarah has been with me on this hair journey right from the very beginning. Sarah and I have been friends for a lifetime. Friends first, we always said we wished we were sisters or cousins. One day that wish came true when a different uncle started to date her mum. We were ecstatic about it at the time, our wishes had come true. Years later, we both laugh and say, "Be careful what you wish for" because that relationship didn't end well at all. However, we are still close, so that's one consolation.

Sarah had always wanted to be a hairdresser, for as long as I could remember and as a child was constantly styling our hairs. From the age of sixteen, she finally started her career, beginning as a trainee. Sarah would always ask me if I would volunteer to be a salon model. The first time she did this, I allowed her to cut my hair. My cousin is white British with European hair, naturally straight and brunette. She had just started her career and without any recognition of the differences between afro and European hair, she asked me if she could practice. Because I was always the kind of person who wanted to see people reach their potential, I let her loose on my hair. Looking all professional, scissors in hand, such a simple task...or so she thought.

At the time, my cousin didn't understand the differences. She started cutting my hair whilst wet and after much snipping and then drying it, she was mortified to find out that afro hair, with its little curls, was a third of the length once dry. So, there I was, looking in the mirror with what appeared to be a one-inch haircut. Obviously apologetic, I must really love her because she's had her hands on my head many times since, even after that nightmare.

I realised, many, many years ago, that there are different types of hair care workers. Firstly, it started with an understanding from my cousin after years of studying, telling me in no uncertain terms that, "I'm not a hairdresser, I'm a stylist'.

This continued for years, where I paid absolutely no attention to her going on at me. This was until I grew up and developed my own career, thus forming a mature respect for people in their chosen craft. I observed her in her practice to understand the difference and gave the relevant respect and credit where it was due. This was most of the time, except one dreaded day when she arrived to visit with vibrant bright red hair. I blurted out my distaste, and to this day, I don't think she has truly forgiven me.

Years later, I met my fantastic hair care specialist who understands hair on a deeper level. Because of this, for the last five years, my hair has been at its best in terms of treatments and timely cutting schedules and first and foremost, because her work has been second to none.

Not only was she responsible for rescuing my hair when I started my menopause, she was also responsible for doing my wedding hair, which was the most fantastic style I had seen in a long time. As soon as the wedding pictures were posted online, it got so much attention on social media that people were constantly asking her if they could have their hair recreated in the same manner. Unfortunately for those soon to be brides, she liked her styles to be unique and had to gently let these eager brides down.

With that being said, I ask myself, if it wasn't for my hair specialist, what would my hair look like now? Following the introduction of the dreaded M-word, without a doubt, my menopause has been detrimental to my lovely locks.

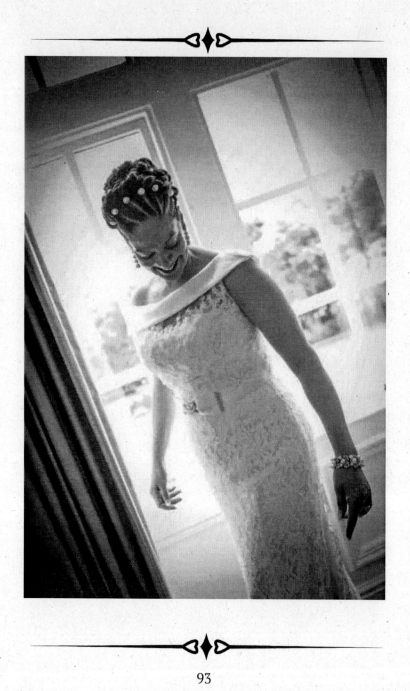

This brings me on to introducing Annie. What can I say about Annie? Well, first, let me say that Annie introduced herself to me, sprouting the most amazing vibrant bright red hair.

I loved it! How things change with age and wisdom.

When she talked about the transition of losing her sacred hair, I could see that this was a very emotional time. Annie described her hair as being so sacred and loved. Now the fact that her beloved hair was falling out brought with it an immense amount of fear.

Before writing the Menopause Diaries, she was a stranger to me. Annie is the kind of lady with one of those beautiful, bountiful spirits. She has the kind of energy after speaking to her for only a few moments which makes you feel like you have known her for years. At fifty-three years young, an Irish woman from Croydon in South London, Annie is an actress and yoga instructor. As Annie beams, she describes all the different platforms where she engages her many skills. From theatrical performing arts and yoga retreats to recently launching her own podcast. I could clearly see that Annie has a lot of pride in the many talents that she delivers to the world.

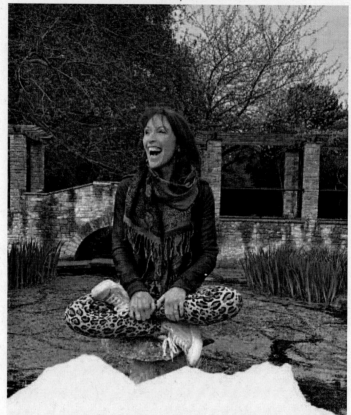

"Talk to your daughters"

ANNIE HAYES-PANTONY

As I interviewed Annie, educating me in her natural teaching style, I learned for the first time that the "actual menopause" was just a one-day celebration. After twelve months of no longer having a period, you are considered as being in menopause. From the next day, you move swiftly on to postmenopause. Annie feels as if the UK societal perception on menopause is that of embarrassment, in her experience.

Annie is now in a good place in terms of accepting and surrendering to this womanly transition, although at the time of the interview, you can still hear the fear and dread in her voice when she talked about this sensitive subject. I've always believed that we tend to have one main fear in life, regarding a collective of experiences as human beings. Although menopause brings a plethora of different symptoms, she experienced sixteen identifiable ones. Hair loss for Annie though, really was the one to dread.

As Annie recounted this experience on the video chat, I wanted to put my arms through the screen and give her a much-needed hug, when she described the painful experience as traumatic. Feeling as though she was already losing her womanhood anyway, the hair loss brought with it new fears. Frightened at the potential outcome of going bald, the hair loss was a tragic experience, to say the least. At the time, turning to HRT to try to counteract this affliction and with no success, Annie decided to stop. However, she did confirm that she would probably give it another try without hesitation if she needed it again. Maybe it's because of my empathetic nature that I could feel the raw pain she must have endured, or perhaps it was because it triggered in me a response to address my own relationship with my hair.

She felt it affected many areas of her life, being known by others playfully as, "Little Red." She found it hard to envisage life without her lovely signature red locks. Annie believes that her natural remedies had some success in making her feel better overall. Her yoga practices were a massive contribution to her feeling as physically well as she does now.

Some of the other symptoms she experienced were heightened emotions, so the hair loss was further compounded due to her emotional state. Admitting that she found more peace when she started working full time for herself, her confidence grew and she began to care less about what others may have thought about it. Finally taking time for herself, she drew from her yoga and stayed grounded. Annie described herself as quite hard, a bit of a tough cookie, and fine-tuned her own coping strategies. Her epiphany came on a trip to Egypt, where she decided that her purpose in life was to share her knowledge of yoga, helping other women in a more meaningful way.

Finding some funny moments, Annie describes when she went out with her partner right at the beginning. Her partner said, "there has been something I have meant to do for ages". In anticipation, Annie thought that he was finally going to tell her that he loved her. She braced herself as he leaned over and plucked a hair from her chin. Although funny, it didn't stop the love from developing, and they continued their journey together. Annie decided that this act must be love, and she calls him her husband today. We wish you all the best, Annie, and many years of love and happiness in this chapter of your life.

It was nice that some of the women I interviewed were able to find some funny moments in their challenging transition. One memory I recall that was not so funny took place when I was at school.

I contracted head lice. Remember when the nit nurse checked your head, and then you would be delivered that dreaded envelope at the end of the day? Well, one day, I got that dreaded envelope. Living with my mum and having the most giant afro, Mum had either no patience or no time to address this issue. I remember my mum cutting all my hair off to about an inch from my scalp to save her the job. I remember not wanting to go back to school and the shame I felt walking in the next day, pondering what my friends would think about me not having my hair. Is this why I forgave my cousin when she did the same thing by accident many years later? Maybe. Had I become numb? Possibly. When women lose their hair, they can feel exposed, or so I'm told.

Since 1997, when I had my first child, I noticed a new hair growth. Up to this point, my hair grew, but never like it did then. My midwife told me it's often the hormone changes that can make your hair, nails, and skin much healthier. Since then and until recently, I have mainly kept my hair long. I started to ask myself why. Was it because some people see long hair as a symbol of youth and beauty? I am told that women hide behind their hair, but was this the case for me? Or was it me making a statement, with a 'now I know I can, so I will' attitude to a world that told me that black girls couldn't have long hair and rebelling against societal perceptions. So many questions have never been explored by me until now. If hair is a symbol of beauty for women and society tells us that black hair is not seen as a classic symbol of beauty, what does actually make us beautiful? Do we have to find another outlet? What do we do?

You already know that I have a beautiful daughter and to date I have spent thousands of pounds letting her have any style that she wants. I don't think there has ever been a time when she said, "Mum, I want to try this," and I said "no".

I have watched over the years as she has tried out the different styles and colours, proud that she has had the confidence to experiment. I always did her hair myself when she was younger. I guess I also tried out different styles on her. Not as elaborate as the skilled hairstylists that she uses now, but I remember once I grew her hair into dreadlocks but decided to take it out after several months. I tirelessly took out each and every lock, one by one, with a fine-tooth comb, careful not to cause her any discomfort. It would have been much easier for me to just cut it off, as suggested by some people. But that was not an option, not after the trauma I faced when my mum did that to me. Funnily enough, only recently she asked to have them put back in. At the time, I wasn't sure if she would appreciate them when she got older, and I felt she was too young to wear something with such deep cultural values without it being her own choice.

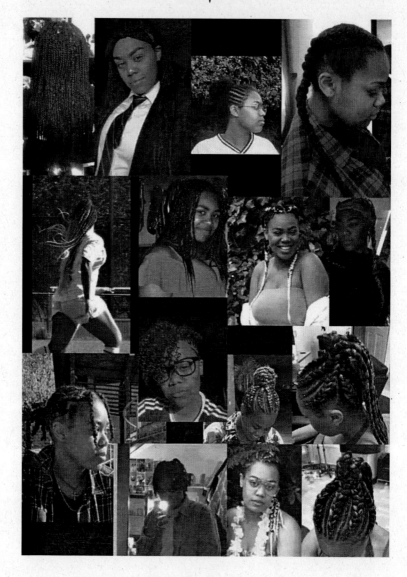

To get some more perspective, I decided to interview Natasha. Natasha is thirty years young and is yet to face menopause. I've known Tasha, as we've nicknamed her, since she was about eight years old. I used to babysit her, alongside her brothers, sisters and cousins. Yes, sometimes there were a lot of children to watch. Tasha having not yet reached menopause, I wanted to know what thoughts went through someone's mind generally about hair and if there were any thoughts about the up-and-coming M saga.

Strangely, as I settled in to talk to her, Natasha admits that as a child, she looked up to me and my hair. I admit that I found this strange. I already knew there were some deeply seated hair issues for her after already admitting this to me recently. Currently embarking on her first business, which is to produce hair care products for afro hair, we had discussed this from a business perspective in my mentor group. I support a group of young adults in their business start-ups. But now, confessing in more detail that she has always struggled to manage and maintain her hair, she admitted that she still struggles today. Tasha says she knows lots of black women who experience this too. Admitting to being confident in most areas of her life, her hair wasn't one of them.

She said that, growing up, she used to look at my hair and wish she had hair like me. In my eyes, my hair was so unmanageable, but Tasha says she used to be in awe of it. She said there is a spectrum of afro hair, and she always wished she had mine. Telling me that she used to think she would grow up one day and it would change to look like mine.

"I remember how confident you were," she says, "and your hair was beautiful." She went on to say that, "The confidence that you had, I believed you could still have had my hair, and I would still have been in awe."

Natasha loved my hair. She wanted my hair and felt that, as an older woman, I had the magical ability to change her hair. Like I said, to me it was strange. As I thought back to that period, it was a time when I used to process my hair a lot, relaxing it at home without guidance. Often seeing it break in different places, I strived to find the beauty I couldn't see but, apparently, others could.

I stopped using chemicals in my hair many years ago, and in my opinion, my hair has never felt more beautiful in its natural state. On reflection, menopause is a natural state of being.

Since my cousin has been with me throughout my whole hair journey, it wouldn't be right not to end this chapter with her appearance. Remember when I told you earlier that I used to wet my hair to tame it as a child? Well, that was only partially true. This ritual went on well into my adult years as well. I can hear my cousin now telling me all the time not to wet my hair, cautioning me that it will all break off. It never stopped me. I kept going because it was already a part of my daily routine.

One day in 2001, my cousin called me and asked me to make time and come to the salon. She wanted to experiment on my hair again. Her employer had succumbed to a new purchase when visited by a sales rep, purchasing some new GHDs. Apparently, as the agent spoke, my cousin said that all that stuck out in her mind as he gave his long hard sales pitch was when he said, "These are so good they will even straighten afro hair."

Sarah has always worked in European salons, so I think it was just her love for me, her cousin, sister and friend, that kept her abnormal interest in my hair plight all these years. She was eager to try them on me, curious if they were true to their word.

My cousin has spent years watching me with my immovable, dense, thick afro, so here we were again. After hours, when the salon closed, the latest experiment was pending as we began. Starting at the hair shaft and slowly gliding out towards the end, she eagerly informed me that it was working on the fourth glide. She toiled away for hours as she enthusiastically worked on my whole head of hair.

Three hours later, she told me she was finished. She allowed me to finally see what she had done. She spun my chair around to face the mirror as she showed me my perfectly straight hair. It was truly perfect. Straight, flowing, and moveable. It was the hair that I had dreamed of all those years ago, sitting in the bath with my bottle of conditioner. Remember when I confessed that I didn't cry very much in Chapter Two? Well, when we looked at each other on this day, we both started to cry. We cried for what seemed like ages. As I looked at myself in the mirror, I felt beautiful for the first time in my life.

So, there it is. The end of this reflective journey. Emotional, to say the least, I have laughed to myself recounting individual stories and I have cried to myself reciting others. Looking back, I figured out that the number of hair stories I have could be a book in and of themselves. Sharing only a few with you this time to try and stay on topic, the realisation I came to was that my hair has always been a thing. I just didn't know it.

The little girl in me realised that my relationship with my hair was broken because I was never given the love and attention that all little girls need. What I had to endure with this lack of love and guidance was traumatic, which led me to build a protective disassociation with my hair. I thought about my actions with my own daughter and how I gave too much because I had so little. I sadly thought of the millions of other sisters who may have gone through similar experiences.

I remembered we were all different. Being a mixed-race woman growing up with a white mother who probably didn't have access to any support or guidance at the time, I chose to believe that this was the case as it was less painful. Thinking about society today and the wealth of information online, which means little girls can access all they need to support them on this journey, I compare it to growing up in the seventies and eighties when we didn't have that.

I thought about the role model I had been to other mixed race little girls even though I was totally unaware. I thought about my role models in the form of my Rastafari Empresses who exuded a powerful confidence that my spirit was drawn to.

I realised that more education was needed, for hairdressers and stylists, so they can understand the complexities of our hair. Happily, my cousin informs me that this is still an ongoing fight but, very soon, afro hair is to be included in the mandatory training. As with most things, it has taken a while, but fingers crossed, at least it is on its way.

I thought about Annie, who is white with European hair with her own pain and struggles. My cousin says it is different for white women, although, in some ways, it is the same. All women have an attachment to their hair. It is the first thing people notice when they see you. If someone contracts cancer and experiences hair loss, a lot of women wear wigs to hide from the world. White women apparently see hair as a symbol of youth, so they will strive to keep that youthful appearance as long as possible.

I end this chapter with an acknowledgement of something that I have never acknowledged. I started by telling you that my hair was never a thing. But it's clear that subconsciously I have thought about it, never at the forefront of my mind, yet hidden deep under the layers of trauma.

It is not a black and white thing. It is a woman thing. We are all our sisters' keepers. When one hurts, so should we all. What we should all remember, as India Arie says, is, "I am not my hair."

Remember and nurture that little girl in you and be sensitive to your daughters. Teach them that they are beautiful and every inch of them matters. If we all do this then no matter the reason they encounter hair loss, they can be empowered and stand strong.

Let us go see about self-care.

From No Hair to Self Care

During the writing of this book, I decided to take a trip to the island of Jamaica. The trip wasn't only to experience the natural beauty that the island has to offer, but to collect my daddy. Stuck inside during the Covid 19 lockdown of 2020, he hadn't really left the house since March 2020 and it was now June 2021. I had a mission to fulfil: to go and spend a few days and then get him safely back to the UK. This brings me quite naturally into this chapter for more than one reason.

Self-care has been high on the agenda for most of the women I have spoken to. It seems as though the journey is less overwhelming and the women can see clearer once they learn about and prioritise self-care. This is from both my own personal experience and most of the women I have spoken to. So, let's start with Jamaica because, as the events of the trip unfolded, they highlighted a significant character trait I think most women have. Or maybe a character flaw would be more apt?

I arrived at Montego Bay Airport. All I could think about was getting to see my dad, as he will be eighty-five on his next birthday. Two years without a 'Daddy hug' was all I could think of. My plane arrived early... result. I walked out into the beautiful sunshine, found myself a seat and waited for my lift to arrive.

Three hot and sweaty hours later, my cousin rolled up giving me some tale about the rain slowing him down, with actual video evidence to back up his story. I joked with him that if he had set off in time, the rain wouldn't have been the problem, playfully teasing him that the rain was karma teaching him a lesson. I love my cousin with his big infectious smile.

My menopause was happy and chilled because it was warm, luckily for me the hot flushes were kept at bay. Anyone who knows me is aware of how much a bit of sun can make my day. We headed off on the next three-hour leg of the journey. I've already mentioned before that all this was due to the second dreaded C word - Covid - and now my dad was ready to come home. The only issue was that he was still quite scared and would not travel alone. Therefore, I was happy to step in as his personal chaperone.

Since I was already writing this book, I figured it would give me a brilliant opportunity to continue my work for a few days with pleasant surroundings and in peace away from my usual life demands.

After a long flight and a bumpy drive back from the airport, stopping only to eat curried goat and rice, we pulled up outside the house. I felt excited as I anticipated feelings of home. When my dad appeared on the porch, wearing a beaming smile, instantly I felt at peace. After our socially distanced greetings and managing to settle my racing heart, I settled into my room, unpacked my bags and spent a little bit of time catching up.

At first glance, it was apparent that my dad had taken time to prepare the house for his new long-awaited guest. As I spent more time looking around, I noticed a few worrying signs highlighting a lack of self-care.

I've already mentioned that my dad will be eighty-five years young on his next birthday. He is pretty healthy for his age and fully self-sufficient. His house was very tidy, but a couple of areas were dirty and in need of a little 'TLC'.

More worryingly, I noticed that my dad had issues with his gas boiler in the bathroom. It had been blowing black smoke up to the ceiling and around the walls. My heart sank as thoughts raced through my mind, thinking every 'what if' possible. I was terrified for my dad, a man who was so fiercely independent and equally strong-willed as his daughter. So, after speaking to him for a few moments, ever so gently discussing my observations, my dad said that he was waiting for this pandemic to be over so that he could restock his cleaning supplies. He had run out but did not want to bother anybody. My dad has always been like this and I don't know if it is cultural or generational but Dad tends to avoid asking for help. I felt distraught but made sure that I didn't show my true feelings. It was clear that Dad had made so much effort to ensure I was welcomed with a nice place to stay.

My dad is my king. I have mentioned previously that, as a child, I suffered different forms of abuse. Just for point of reference, none of it came from his side. My dad has always strived hard to ensure that his children were well looked after, but unfortunately, when you are caught up in a custody battle, these things are sometimes taken out of your hands.

The following day, I broke my quarantine and popped into the local shop, which is literally five hundred meters up the road. I bought all the bleach, cloths and multi-purpose cleaner that my rucksack could hold, filling an additional beach bag with more cleaning supplies. In my hands, I carried new shower curtains, a soap rack and a bathmat.

I returned to the house, a lady on a mission. I told Dad that I would spend the next couple of days cleaning everything and getting it back up to scratch, reminding him that I also appreciated the apparent effort he had definitely made for my arrival. A different cousin popped around to have a garden visit, bringing his wife and my auntie Lurline with him. I quietly pulled him to one side, and donning masks, we went to look at the boiler.

My cousin and I hatched a plan to redo the bathroom and install a wet room whilst my dad and I were visiting the UK. I also showed him a couple of areas that needed some bleach. My cousin obviously felt terrible but I reassured him, as I know how scared my dad has been throughout this pandemic. Not wanting any visitors inside the house, I asked my cousin to ask Dad to step outside in future while he does a little check around.

You might ask how this relates to self-care? Self-care is looking after oneself without always prioritising the needs of others. My dad felt like he did not want to be a burden, and I'm sure that he would not have been in the slightest. This stopped him from asking for what he needed for fear of putting others out. It pains me because I know that my Jamaican family are the most loving and supportive type. I wish my dad had been clear about his needs so that they could have been met. I know that the scenario I'm referencing is not directly related to menopause but what accomplishment of mine would be complete without a guest appearance of the leading man, Daddy G.

More importantly, the scenario highlights that we all need to look after ourselves. I find it fascinating from interviewing all these extraordinary women and through my own reflections on the menopausal journey, that self-care is fundamentally one of the most essential tools which can help women through this transition.

As women, we go through most of our lives thinking of others first, either raising children, looking after parents, or emotionally supporting others. We are the first to offer to make cookies and cakes for a school event or offer to babysit for a friend. We nurture those around us, and we think emotionally without always giving practicalities a second thought.

Since being ten years old, I have worked, starting with the usual paper round and working my way up. By the age of twelve, I worked in an ice cream factory on the weekend, both Saturdays and Sundays doing eight-hour shifts. My brother and I had told a little lie and said that we were sixteen-year-old twins when, in fact, I was twelve and he was fourteen years old.

Note that this wasn't legal at the time and my brother and I didn't have national insurance numbers to make it a long-term project. Every weekend we were asked for the national insurance number by our boss and we just kept making excuses for why we kept forgetting it. If memory serves me, I think we earned around thirty pounds a day, which was a tidy sum back then, especially for a twelve-year-old.

I remember the reason I did this was that I liked feeling independent. I wanted to save and buy my own clothes and didn't want to continue to burden my parents. I don't think these days you would get away with that for more than a few weeks but, back then, this went on for several months, earning us a tidy packet. I prefer not to focus on the lies I told back then, but to celebrate the entrepreneurial spirit instead.

My son has a personality similar to mine; straight talking, inquisitive and abundantly passionate. Constantly going on at me for giving money away to strangers, he thinks that it only fuels people to buy drugs if they have a habit, but it really etches a dark feeling on my soul if I walk past someone who appears less fortunate than me. I will often purchase meals or give people money in their hands as I feel it is not my place to judge them.

More often than not, as women, we host parties and take responsibility for keeping families together. We are the first to think about adoption and fostering either orphaned animals or children. We tend to work in charitable or voluntary sectors supporting those in need. I have worked in a sector for eleven years now, where the financial rewards are minimal, but the social gains are enormous. I am often told I could have made much more money with my strong personality and savvy ways if I had done something else in a more cut-throat sector. I don't mind those who choose to judge me, not that it matters, but I have my fingers in several pies anyway. There is this strange concept that some people feel the need to work out other people's lives. I personally see this as a total waste of energy. That energy is always best used to work on your own path and your own development.

Having said all that, when it came to this chapter of my life, the realisation was that it was time to think of me first. It started during the year of the 2020 pandemic, when both my children raised concerns about me. One day while sitting outside in the sun, ignoring the dreaded ivy that was imposing itself around the whole third quarter of my garden, my son turned to me bluntly telling me that he felt I was "letting myself go." In fact, both of my children said they were worried and gave me a 'tough-love' talk. They were unaware how perfect the timing was as I had recently been reflecting on this myself, especially in relation to my marriage.

Through these conversations, I was able to look thoroughly at my emotions and how I had slipped into this dark place. One where I was literally going through the motions of the day but not feeling anything, numb to the issues that were going on around me, this new scary place. Yes, I'm talking about my menopause and the lonely marriage that I had somehow found myself in. I had to place myself in a vulnerable position and allow my children to discuss their observations with me, openly and transparently, forcing myself to listen to things that were painful to hear.

It was deep, but with it came a new understanding of the place that I had arrived and they, my children, my babies, were allowed a platform of healing provided by me. With it came a further evolution of growth within our relationships and lives.

It's tough when those words come from your own children, one of which was still a minor. My daughter, unlike my son, is known famously within the family as "the quiet one". She was only fifteen years old at the time. She is the kind of person who, when she speaks, you hear her because she doesn't speak that much. She may still have to fight to be heard some days, but that's a work in progress. I thank them both because this sort of tough love is what got me out of a rut that I, for the most part, wasn't even aware I was in. Was it a process? Yes, it was. Was it easy? No, it was not. I had to dig deep, reflect, surrender and have some tough open conversations with myself and those around me whom I love.

I have always been very close with them both but don't get me wrong, we have our moments as most parents do. It was with warmth and sensitivity they brought these matters to my attention. I decided I could not ignore their cries. It felt familiar, much like that of a parent to a child and similar to the feelings I felt towards my dad. I knew I needed to act. My plans evolved and became more focussed over time. Initially, I wouldn't say that I had a goal per se, but I definitely had bullet points of things that needed to change and fast.

Some of these things were to start moving again, just getting out in the day, going for a walk, and doing regular everyday things like gardening.

Another was to start thinking of myself first, as my children quite rightly reminded me, I have spent many years giving myself to others, be it in my job as a homecare manager, supporting my staff, or supporting my friends, my first husband, second husband and the partners in between. I'm a giver and my children know that, but my children had to tell me to stop.

My children reminded me that I should be the only one who matters right now. They reminded me that I'm no good to anyone if I'm no good to myself. They reminded me how much they loved me.

The most poignant message I took from the discussions was that they have always loved and depended on me. Right now, they were worried because I was not that 'strong person' they had come to know and love. They said they wanted me to look after myself, starting straightaway, they wanted me to return to the person who made them feel safe and getting back on track to being around for a long time. Cue the tears from the tough-love talk. They were right and as the words dropped out of their mouths, I started to reflect on my current situation, realising I had forgotten the most important person. I had forgotten about me.

Who was I, and what did I want for my future?

A third point was to focus on my diet. I was currently eating anything and everything; not necessarily too much food, but definitely not the right foods and at the wrong time of day. I was fuelling my body with nothing that could be remotely considered nutritious.

And finally, the last thing on my list was to go back and remember things that I truly enjoyed. Something that over the years, I had either put on the back burner, forgotten about or placed so low on my list of priorities that I just never allocated any time.

Ironically, I went back to some of my childhood dreams, one of which was being an artist and another was being a writer. It was my son who actually connected the dots one day. Out of the blue as I was working on a chapter of this book, he asked me what I wanted to do when I was younger. And when I told him, he laughed and said, "funny that isn't it, look at what you're doing right now!"

So, what did I start to do to turn things around? Well, this was the fun part. I love nature and it was the start of lockdown. I built the beautiful garden as previously mentioned. It was demanding and strenuous work, but definitely worth it. I made a conscious effort to spend time every day around nature, even if it was only for a few minutes a day.

I started reading again. I read at least a book a week in my younger years, which sadly became one or two in the last decade.

I'm currently reading a book called "Sacred Self-Care Everyday rituals for a more joyful and meaningful life" written by Chloe Isidora. Two of my staff lovingly gifted it for my birthday, and it couldn't have come at a better time.

I started to meditate daily after putting together a beautiful meditation corner in my lounge. I believe that meditation truly helps with any stress levels that I may be having, whether consciously or subconsciously.

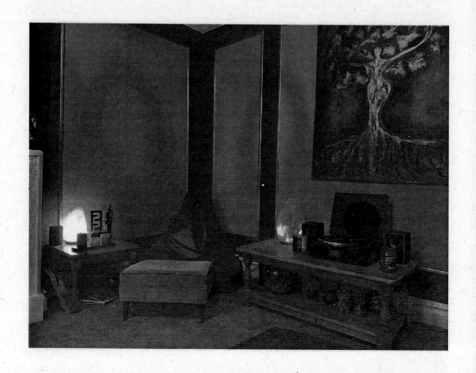

Listening to music had always been a passion of mine and it became a part of everyday life again. I remembered the power of music and installed Alexa into every room in the house so that no matter where I was or what I was doing, I could get a good vibe going on demand.

I reached out and found support on social media platforms. I was never one to be hung up on these platforms before. Now I believe that with the proper focus and discipline, they can be a fantastic support tool.

As I mentioned previously, I started eating better and not so much in quantity. I started eating to live, not living to eat and I kept reminding myself of a funny little saying my cousin used to tell me in the past: "It's food, not love."

I was now making sure that I ate food that would nourish me and not just because I was hungry.

I get regular blood tests to make sure that my vitamins and minerals are at the proper levels.

I had a massive shift in attitude and turned into Frank Sinatra and decided I'd do it 'My Way'. I changed my whole frame of thinking and turned the focus onto me.

Finally, I focussed on working on those relationships that truly matter. I spent time making all my interactions as meaningful as I could. Even when things didn't go to plan, I consciously made an effort to reflect and grow, not taking things to heart and not allowing anyone to disturb my inner peace, no matter what.

Now enough about me, let's look at another scary symptom that one of our ladies experienced. Not one on my own personal list, but terrifying to say the least.

Let us meet Caterina, who is fifty-two years young. Before home-educating her amazingly bright daughter, she worked as a nursery manager and before this, a deputy nursery manager. Coming from Yorkshire in England, Caterina has resided in Australia for the last fourteen years. I came to know Caterina through my children attending her nursery.

Firstly, I thank Caterina for leaving me with a sense of safety to pursue my dreams. She always made me feel like my children were in the best of hands, giving me the peace of mind that all parents need. She enabled me, a single working mum at the time, to pursue my dreams at university then my chosen career. First and foremost, I am genuinely grateful.

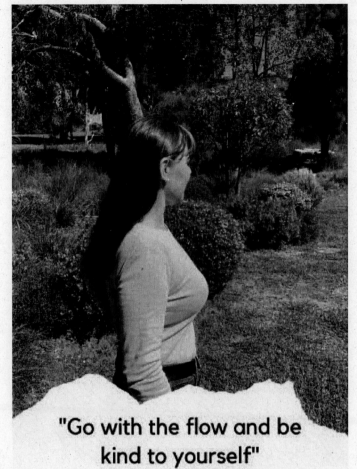

"Go with the flow and be
kind to yourself"

CATERINA GATENBY

So, here's Caterina's story. How has this transition impacted her life? My first observation when interviewing Caterina was that at least half of the interview was taken up with Caterina talking with great pride about her husband and daughter. It was so moving to hear but fits appropriately into the points I'm trying to make. Now, I'm not saying that she doesn't understand her self-care at this point in life, but it is apparent that she has the needs of others high on her priority list.

Home-educating her young daughter while working through her menopause, she was aware that there were three stages, but not sure what defined them all. Caterina did have some understanding and was aware of the symptoms as they crept into her life. She began to experience irregular periods, hot flushes at night (night sweats) and endured some disturbed sleep. Caterina experienced a total of twelve identifiable symptoms. In the same breath, Caterina was also starting to experience a deterioration in her eyesight, which was familiar to her because this indicated a sign of old age within her family. She therefore attributed the other symptoms that she was experiencing at the time, to the same onset of old age.

Caterina went on a cruise around three years ago. The trip was meant to be the holiday of a lifetime, a magical experience for Caterina, her husband and their daughter who had always dreamt of going on a cruise after watching a documentary. At eight years old, her daughter had set up her own business selling greeting cards and spent a year saving up, in true entrepreneurial spirit.

What was meant to be a dream come true was in fact, "a holiday from hell". The experience was far from dream-like. Ranging from inconsiderate hosts who refused to allow this amazing child to dance at a gala after she designed her own amazing outfit, to sending her a letter demanding a credit card despite only being a child.

As Caterina describes, there were so many things that added to the discomfort. Starting to feel pain in her chest shortly after the cruise ended and with elevated stress levels, she found herself attending a hospital visit.

Talking me through the incident, it's as though Caterina almost apologised for causing her family any inconvenience. Whilst in hospital, unable to determine the cause of the chest pains, she was asked about menopause. Realising that this was something she hadn't thought much about before, Caterina's symptoms were then placed at the forefront of her mind.

Afterwards, Caterina reflected on the raised stress levels. She wondered if menopause added to her inability to deal with the situation successfully. After many years of experience dealing with high pressure jobs, she found it unusual. Pain and palpitations were the order of the day, something we haven't talked much about as of yet. From the few women I have spoken to about this, heart palpitations can be a terrifying phenomenon. Your heart starts to race, and some women compare it to feeling like they are having a heart attack.

Caterina reminisces about her mum's menopause, saying that her mum got "a bit hot" at the time but didn't take anything for it. Caterina remembers asking her if she was going to get something to help. Her response was, "Well, no, this is what life is. It's like being a teenager, only at the other end."

This shaped Caterina's outlook on what to expect. Getting the same misinformation from her manager as well, some years earlier in her job, she felt as though it was something that should not be spoken about in the UK unless between close friends. As a manager of an older group of female employees, Caterina had previously offered support to her staff, allowing staff to go home on occasions if they were struggling at work.

Recounting her experiences, her attitude was that, up until now, she put most of her symptoms down to life experience and the stresses of home schooling a child with special needs. Admitting that she may have been wrong, she hasn't linked any of it to her menopause. She did add that following our interview, maybe she should have.

She decided not to take HRT. Two women that Caterina knows have both developed breast cancer, which influenced her decision. She wasn't sure if HRT was directly responsible, so she only took natural supplements in the form of herbal teas, which she feels helped her manage.

Brain fog has caused some of the funniest situations that Caterina has experienced. Although not being able to think of any of her amusing stories in the moment, she did share a funny story about a friend who at one time lost her pants and later found them in the fridge.

Recently in the car, unable to think of a word whilst chatting to her husband, he very patiently reminded her of it after giving her time to think. Caterina has had lots of support from her partner, who has been emotionally sensitive to her experiences. When asked if Caterina consciously finds time for herself, she laughs and says, "Where would I have the time?"

It is vital that we all make time for ourselves. I hope that you get to this point of understanding, my dear sister, Caterina. You are such an amazing mother. Look after yourself so that you can be strong for others. You are important too.

Lynsey is our next sister who, unlike Caterina, was able to swiftly apply important changes that allowed her to put herself first.

Lynsey was one of my childhood friends and is currently forty-seven years young. Having lost contact for several years, we recently spent a bit of time together. Lynsey supported our company, working for me during the pandemic whilst furloughed from her main job. She was as funny and level-headed as I remember, it was lovely having her around for almost a year. I remember Lynsey fanning herself regularly during this time as she mirrored me with my hot flushes. It never stopped her, however, from immersing herself fully into the role to provide a thorough service to our clients.

Currently, in her perimenopause, Lynsey has experienced symptoms since she was forty-one. Not knowing that she was entering menopause, she recalls getting a variety of minor illnesses at the time. Experiencing small bouts of feeling tired, or suffering headaches, she said she experienced nothing major.

When she became anaemic and started to notice bruising that didn't heal, Lynsey finally attended the doctor. After testing her blood, the nurse confirmed that she was in her perimenopause. Asking the nurse about the perimenopause, having no idea what it was, she got the response, "Well, you're a bit young yet, so we'll discuss it later."

Lynsey didn't want to accept that, so politely demanded that she be informed now. This led the nurse to give her a much more 'in-depth' answer of, "It means you're about to go into menopause."

Recalling the nurse as very dismissive, Lynsey went home and sought comfort from Doctor Google. Her only prior knowledge was basically that your periods stopped, and you could get moody and have hot sweats.

Living in the UK, Lynsey feels that the version of menopause taught to people is that it's an age thing and simply signifies that you are getting old.

Experiencing seventeen identifiable symptoms, she laughs at the mention of an increase in irritability, admitting that she could get irritable over the slightest things; something she would be unaware of if her husband didn't point it out. She states that she also developed hay fever for the first time in her life, which I have also heard from a few of our ladies. Admitting that although she could identify the symptoms discussed in the interview, she didn't always make the connection to menopause.

Lynsey took a couple of natural remedies when the symptoms became unmanageable but is currently not taking anything as she says that all is okay. In the beginning, she experienced heightened emotions, even crying at the news, or going to sleep thinking about issues in the world. The thought of children suffering in war-torn countries could wake her up at night; she would get online and donate to charities. Most of us are familiar with this, I call it the witching hour between 3am and 6am when you just cannot sleep.

Lynsey had a terrifying time when her mum was diagnosed with dementia. Lynsey knew that the Dementia was induced by a poor lifestyle. Knowing this, she cried for the whole day, feeling scared that she would go down the same path after watching something on the television.

Lynsey admits that the menopause made her feel weak. She realised that she was the strong one in the family, and she had to look after everyone stating, "I don't have time to be weak."

This helped Lynsey to take more care of herself. She started going to the gym and becoming more active.

Lynsey recalls a time when she attended a children's party. Her love of bouncy castles and passionate personality meant that she couldn't pass on the opportunity to join in with the kids and have some fun. Unfortunately, Lynsey bounced up and down and actually wet her pants. Not a little dribble, but a full-on soaking. Feeling it running down her leg, she jumped off quickly to regain some form of dignity and spent the rest of the day walking around in a pair of jeans that were two sizes too small.

Not receiving any helpful advice from anyone, in all the time that she has endured the trials, she says all the information she has ever received was always negative and not very useful.

Lynsey also admits that she is very conscious of never doing star jumps on her visits to the gym. Her most poignant advice is that it's helpful to find the information about the symptoms and see the funny side.

"It's not all bad," she says. "We will all get through it together."

At the interview's closing, Lynsey thanked me for opening her eyes to an array of symptoms that she wasn't aware of. She said it made her feel as though she had just had some therapy and felt much better. I'm glad for you, young lady... It's always a pleasure to be in your presence.

When speaking to our Queens, I've noticed that some reach this epiphany earlier on. Some get there eventually, and some are still yet to find this sense of freedom which I have mentioned.

I believe that every woman will have their own journey, but I can't stress this enough. When my mindset changed, the unimaginable freedom that came from it was mind-blowing. I only hope that all women can find their own sense of freedom as they enter this stage of life.

With the blessing I found from acceptance, finally came my inner peace.

I think that's the second time we have had women bravely disclose that they have wet their pants. Well, bravo and good on you! Oh, and yes, if you're wondering, I have wet mine too!!!

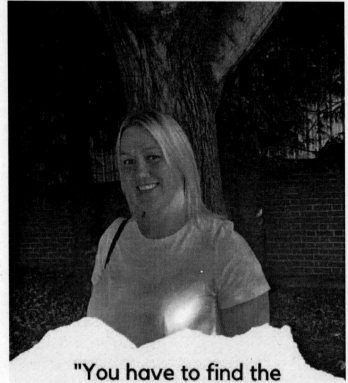

"You have to find the funny side. It's not all bad, we will all get through it together"

LYNSEY ASHWORTH

Reaching the Big M-word

After all of that, I'm finally moving on from perimenopause to explaining the actual Menopause. My trusted doctor (cue laughter and sparkles) confirms that menopause is when you've officially had twelve months without a period.

So, what happens now?

Well, nothing really!

WHAT? I hear you say. The next stage is literally one day, as I was so eloquently informed by our beloved Annie from chapter five.

Menopause means that you have not had a period for twelve months and then you go straight into post-menopause without time for so much as a party!

Well, do you know what ladies? We are not having that! Please, take some time out, go put on your favourite song and dance like no one is watching!

Proceedings will resume momentarily, now go enjoy the moment!!

Menopause V's Man on Pause

Sometimes, when you're in menopause, you turn around, breathe and take stock. You realise that there are all kinds of debris left behind. Looking left, right, front and at the back of you, my goodness it can be everywhere.

We all know that relationships come in all different shapes and sizes. If two women are in a relationship and even one of them started experiencing life-changing emotions, how difficult could that be? And what happens when a woman going through menopause is married to a man who also hits his own mid-life crisis (or as I refer to it, 'man on pause')?

It's like Bonfire Night every single day. I don't mean those pretty fireworks shooting into the sky where you can look into the atmosphere in amazement, mouth open and gob smacked at the array of beauty in the sky. I'm talking about a group of teenagers who illegally bought fireworks from the corner shop, and they are shooting them for fun around the streets.

You're ducking, diving, twisting and turning in and out of backstreets trying to stay out of the way of these rockets, for fear of your life. When you're constantly running from these monsters chasing you, the beast being the symptoms of your situation.

Before I introduce another of our sisters to you, let me tell you first about my experience.

It was June 2016. I remember the day but only vaguely. The thing I do remember is what a beautiful wedding it was. In fairness, most people told me over the years that a wedding can be a blur. The after-effects are almost dreamlike because of the excitement and adrenaline on the day. I had the same experience with my first wedding, but that's a whole different story.

The truth is that on the day I got married to my second husband, I was in the middle of a personal trauma. Unfortunately, my son had gone on vacation, at Her Majesty's request. He was incarcerated for only a few months, but I spent a few years in a semi coma-like state. I knew that my mind wasn't in the right place and I tried to postpone the wedding.

When I look back now, I remember my husband telling me that we should not do that. He convinced me that the time was now. For those of you who have children, I am sure that you can understand what I am going to say. Having your motherhood taken away is the most excruciating pain that a woman can go through. As a mother, your instinct is to rescue your child from the pains of the world. I know that my sisters who don't have children can relate too. Not being able to save my son from this bad situation is the hardest thing I've ever had to endure in my life.

Like I said, I remember the wedding being incredibly beautiful, but then I am the kind of woman who always strives to achieve great things. So, in the midst of my coma, I bucked up and created the wedding every little girl dreams of.

Even to this day, I have not met one guest who hasn't told me what an amazing day it was. People revelled in the beautiful location, amazed at the detail and intricate design links that reflected both of our personalities. They talk about how much laughter and love was in the room and how amazing they felt in the presence of such devotion. I now wonder whether the devotion wasn't so much to each other as to the feeling of being happy.

At the point of getting married, I'd known my second husband for many years as an acquaintance. In passing, he was always polite and friendly, but in 2014 we connected on a different level, there was a different energy and vibe. All relationships have a honeymoon period as you are getting to know each other, sharing stories and sharing each other's dreams.

He's funny and I love to laugh. I'm accomplished and I don't say that arrogantly; I just say it in my truth. To this day, I know wholeheartedly that the only thing I truly wanted in any partnership was someone I could connect with on an emotional level, a person to share my life with and to feel as though I was worth loving. I guess we all have a specific vision for where our lives need to be. Never striving to be a millionaire, I just strived to be self-sufficient. When my second husband and I connected, I was established so I wanted for nothing more now. Or so I thought.

My second husband is an amazing musician, and when I say amazing, he really is. He has a talent that most musicians can only dream of having. You could say that he was born to play. I figured that when I met him through our love of music, his thoughtfulness and the fact that he can be so funny would be enough. But the truth is that every human being on this planet has their own pain and trauma hidden in the depths of their soul. Unfortunately, relationships are where they decide to come out and play.

So here I was, married for the second time, in the midst of my own personal struggles and moving into menopause. My thoughts were consumed with my son and the direction his life had taken. I believe that my second husband hit his own midlife crisis shortly after. This really didn't play out well.

I remember a time when he was in awe and I remember how proudly he used to talk to people about everything I had achieved. However, during our engagement period, I was so preoccupied with my own wants and needs that I missed the signs of his achievements, or lack thereof. I know now that I was his enabler and people only do to you what you allow them to, don't they?

I guess I had been numb to the problems, living in my semi coma-like state. There were many issues, but I was just not paying attention, or not giving them the attention that they deserved.

Coming out of my coma-like state following the tough love talk from my children, I knew that it was make-or-break time. Thinking about the relationship in detail, recalling the last few years, I realised that most of it was a blur.

As I meditated on the experience, I realised that since our energies entwined in 2014 it had been almost seven years so far. I remembered being ecstatically happy for the first eighteen months and then little by little, small concerns started to show their face. We had issues with countless things moving forward.

The first one that raised its head was his lack of drive. Fast forward and the arguing started regularly. The intimacy became less and less frequent. I felt starved, deprived of something that I feel is a basic human need. Intimacy isn't just about sex, it's about a connection of spirits and an intertwining of souls. I am such a tactile person so I really didn't like the place we had reached.

People were starting to notice. One day, when my first husband was over from America visiting his daughter, he pulled me to one side and said, "Can I ask you something? I don't want you to take this the wrong way, but what does your husband do?"

He continued, "I have been here all week and I haven't even seen him take out the garbage."

I couldn't get his words out of my mind. I pondered what he had said. It was true, my second husband didn't do a thing. He didn't wash, cook or shop. He didn't pay any bills, organise anything for the family or book holidays. He didn't initiate conversations or do things with the kids. He did absolutely nothing. I thought about it for a long time, wondering how I could have been with someone for so long, who contributed nothing at all.

I realised eventually that it was because I truly am self-sufficient. I have always been proactive, so I continued to take care of business and I guess he just got comfy with being taken care of.

When I was having the tough love talk from the kids, which followed shortly after, they said pretty much the same. Coming from my kids, I heard it more. They didn't hold back. They lived with me, so their observations were thorough and deep.

Fast forward to June 2021, my husband and I decided to give it another go. Actually, let me correct myself, it was I who decided to give it another go and brought the suggestion to him. My soft nature got the better of me. I had justified all my husband's actions in my mind. I reasoned that he must be allowing parts of his own journey to dictate his behaviour. He had told me things about his own journey in the past, times when he himself had experienced pain.

Maybe these were the same experiences that he was allowing to creep into our relationship and they were now affecting his connection with me? It was to my children's dismay, but I've said it already, they who feel it know. My children, and others for that matter, who haven't experienced the magnitude of changes that a woman goes through with menopause, would always find it difficult to understand.

As with most relationships, we have a tendency of looking too deeply at the situation, reasoning the why and the what of the experience.

At this point, I had done enough reflecting on myself and our relationship to know that not all the fault lay with my second husband. I had to take ownership of the changes that I had come through and the reactions I might have had due to these changes.

I also had to be honest and admit that my son being taken away prevented me from being fully present for a time, I was distracted and distant. I had to own my menopause and at times I had allowed it to take over my mind and body, causing me to become impatient and emotional.

One thing I did know was that I had transitioned into a different stage in life. I was another person to the one my husband connected with in 2014. Please don't get me wrong, I am not apologising, but I feel this is where the problems arose. I am human and I have an expectation that my life partner presents an understanding for the experiences that I can and will go through. But he is also a human being, with his own journey and sometimes these journeys are out of balance.

We have all heard the saying "When you are weak then I'll be strong."

But what happens when both are weak at the same time?

I started by talking to my husband the day after our anniversary. I decided that it would be more productive to go away for the night, away from familiar surroundings, a neutral space for us both. I booked us into a beautiful hotel not far from home. We went to have an excellent Thai massage, afternoon tea and an exquisite three-course meal.

The next day we went for a walk in a local nature reserve and we talked. It wasn't easy but I managed to gently encourage him to open up. I made my expectations as a wife very clear and I made it clear that my husband was responsible for presenting his own expectations.

Instead of listing the different things that I wanted to see, I asked my husband to tell me what a good husband looks like in his eyes. I asked him to share with me his experiences and the role that he sees himself in. This didn't appear to come easily to him, which had become the norm. In the past I remember we used to talk for hours and hours at a time, sometimes throughout the whole night. Now it seemed that every conversation was a strain and over time we had become more and more lost for words.

I came away still not very clear. I reminded him that I am entirely self-sufficient financially and I have never needed him to be the so-called breadwinner. I reminded him that I fell in love with him because of our shared love of music, the humour and because he made me feel safe and loved, something I hadn't felt in a long time.

I made sure he was fully aware that the expectations were minimal, as they always had been, but he was still not hitting the mark. I reminded him that nothing had changed in relation to my expectations in the beginning and that I couldn't understand why, when I needed so little, he couldn't even give me that? So again, he made a few excuses for why he hadn't been present. As usual, the excuses were different this time. They always were. Could it be that we'd overcome our troubles and find a way to be happy and grow old, together?

Two weeks later, he made me two cups of tea and gave me two kisses on the cheek. I was done.

And there it was. He walked away; his arms laden with suitcases. Seven years and not even a goodbye. No 'I'm sorry' and no 'Thank you'.

To my husband, I say this. Four years living your life on pause due to your own male issues. Not shining in your own light, unaware of your unique gifts and talent, crippled by your own trauma and pain. Right now, I don't have any more time for pause. I'm working on me. We all need to be ready to change and grow before anyone else can assist us. So, for now, I wish you love and light.

What will happen? I don't really know. What I do know is right now, I'm living in the final chapter of my life. It may be another week, a month or it could be another forty to sixty years of living. Who knows? But I am happy. I'm going to continue to make it my best life, a life by my design, because life is beautiful. It's incredible and deep and rich. Life is seductive with all its possibilities, and I'm ready to continue to seduce it and be seduced by it. Playing out every hope and dream, my dreams that can only be limited by my own imagination.

Did I ever tell you that on my wedding day, I could only get one contact lens in my eye? Could this have been the universe trying to tell me something?

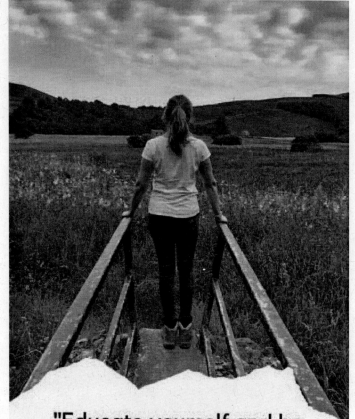

"Educate yourself and be
informed"

NICOLA JANE GIFFORD

Now let's meet Nicola. Like me, she experienced issues with her marriage. At fifty-three years young, born in Scotland and living in England most of her life, Nicola has worked all the way through her menopause as a solicitor.

Forty-six when her symptoms first started, she was unable to accurately pinpoint her periods ending due to the coil. Anxiety, joint pains, a lack of confidence leading to isolation and the inability to face people and an intolerance to alcohol all hit Nicola at the same time.

Nicola did lots of research to ensure that she was informed as she knew very little prior to her symptoms starting, which really helped. At the time, Nicola felt it was pretty taboo but she now feels it is getting better. Nicola feels being in her menopause and actively seeking information about it has improved her experience. It could still be much better, but the light at the end of the tunnel is on its way.

Experiencing eighteen recognisable symptoms, Nicola smiles as she hears me ask if she has experienced irritability.

Not taking HRT in the beginning, Nicola instead opted for herbal remedies such as sage and mood relief tablets, which she admits helped. She stopped working after a year when she decided to go to HRT, which worked very well. Nicola had a good experience with her GP who, I'm happy to tell you, was also male.

During this stage, she sadly recalls that her husband had an affair and left the family home. Nicola feels, without a shadow of a doubt, there are clear links to the end of her marriage and menopause. Often trying to engage him in conversation and make him aware of the struggles she was going through, she felt this was a losing battle. Despite bringing home leaflets and presenting websites to read, Nicola says her attempts fell on deaf ears as he didn't feel like menopause was a real thing. Twenty-eight years of marriage came to an end and Nicola was left on her own. Nicola feels that she is unable to discuss it with her two teenage sons as they are embarrassed to talk about it.

At a particularly emotional stage, Nicola says she felt unable to do her job anymore after she gave a joint presentation at work and literally fell to pieces, only managing to get through it because she was carried by her colleague. Feeling as though she was not performing for the team, she started questioning her own abilities, which left her feeling anxious about being replaced by a younger, more ambitious colleague.

Even though Nicola was aware she was in menopause, she still couldn't seem to control her anxious thoughts. When interviewed, she was unable to recount any funny moments, even in hindsight, she said she found nothing funny at all.

Nicola sadly admitted to having suicidal thoughts at least once or twice. When driving home from work one day, she actually thought about driving her car off a cliff. Scared at that moment, she questioned her whole life, initially reasoning with herself that her children would be better off without her. Telling herself that her life was over anyway, convinced she was no longer a good mother and no longer good at her job.

Looking back, she feels that it was only thoughts of her children that stopped her. Even though her menopausal thoughts made her feel like a failure as a mum, her motherly instincts won the battle and finally snapped her mind back into some form of sensible state.

Within five or six days of taking HRT, Nicola said that she was able to find herself again. Even though her journey meant that previously she wasn't someone who took medication, HRT was a life saver for her. Nicola has happily got her confidence back and is settling into the life that she is designing.

At the time, feeling like a shadow of her former self, she advised me that as women we spend most of our lives looking after others.

"But look after yourself," she says. "Don't be swayed by others and make choices for yourself because, after all, you must live with yourself all the time, and you are the only constant in your own life. I finally did it for me because I wanted to feel like the old me again. I wanted the bouncy vibrant me back. Be selfish and just look after you."

As if to drive her point home, Nicola shows off the bright pink trousers she is wearing for her interview.

"The last chapter in our life is for us, and I'm all over it."

Nicola is ready to live her best life. Wearing those trousers with pride is a statement that she can and will do whatever she wishes.

We could all take a leaf out of your book, Nicola, we wish you all the best with your new found inner strength.

As I mentioned earlier, if menopause met menopause instead of "man on pause" would that cause different issues? Or would there be more of a shared understanding? I decided to talk with Margie to ask her to share her experience of living with her partner during her menopause transition.

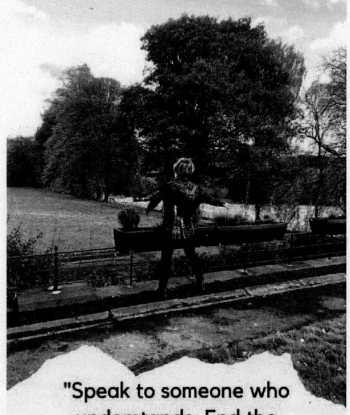

"Speak to someone who understands. End the suffering earlier and please don't live in denial"

MARGIE DE SOUSA

Margie is sixty-two years young. Originally from Portugal before moving to South Africa due to the political unrest and recession at the age of nine, she then settled in the UK over twenty years ago.

Over the moon that we are writing this book and raising awareness of women's menopause struggles, she admits that she has had a rough time. As a hairstylist (not a hairdresser), she attends to many mature ladies and that confirms it is a topic not spoken about freely.

Working through her menopause, which started when she was about forty-eight years old, she is now in post-menopause.

At the time, she recognised that she had transitioned into menopause but admitted to living in denial for some time. In her mind, like many others, menopause was a sign of old age and she wasn't ready to admit that. In a relationship and failing to accept the transition, Margie admits that she behaved in an extreme manner, subsequently breaking up with her partner of seven years. She felt driven, in her words, to "Have a blow-out."

People around her were urging her to seek confirmation from a doctor but Margie had other ideas, choosing to live in total denial.

Being aware that menopause existed, she admitted that she hadn't wanted to look it up because she didn't want to accept the fact. She didn't really understand it. Margie knew that you lost your sex drive, your periods stopped (which would have been a bonus) but that was where her understanding ended.

A part of Margie's thought process was that if she ignored it, it just wasn't there. Obviously, this didn't work out because the symptoms are still there as she describes the hot flushes alongside experiencing nine other recognisable symptoms in total.

Margie states that, in the past, she was always about twelve years older than her peer group. So, when her menopause started, she didn't have a support network. Having friends who have now caught up with her, she is able to broach these discussions and they support each other.

Trying HRT for three months helped to reduce her symptoms, but it didn't agree with her overall, so she stopped. She then started taking various vitamins to assist her, but she has subsequently stopped these too.

One long term partner that Margie met whilst she was in her perimenopause, was herself in menopause. Margie moved away from her home town of Leeds to Brighton and this relationship lasted nine years.

Some of the most poignant memories Margie has are linked with emotions, she recalls becoming very emotional at things, admitting that she still has those experiences even today. Switching from a happy-go-lucky person to almost suicidal, she suffered extreme mood swings. Admitting to becoming very fiery,

Margie describes attending a birthday meal with her friends where everyone was having a great time, but Margie just got up and walked out. Margie felt as if her head was gone. Between the age of fifty and fifty-five, she didn't feel happy with anything, lashing out at her friends for no apparent reason. Margie is grateful that they are still around now she has got over the worst of it.

Having a very positive go-getter attitude, Margie was all good on a superficial level. "Even though you're not getting enough sleep and your body is experiencing this trauma, you still have to function on a day-to-day level" she says. Then, Margie felt her life spiralling.

After a while, she decided to try to regain her life by ending her current relationship, which had now turned into a friendship. Following the loss of both of their sex drives, they were living together with no real intimacy. Margie puts this down to her menopause and her partner being older than her at the time.

Margie doesn't feel as though she would have survived menopause if she didn't make these drastic changes. She felt that she needed to change her mindset and reconnect with her family in Leeds.

Moving back home without a place to stay and no money, Margie admits that when she met her partner, she thought it was going to be a person she would stay with for the rest of her life. This was the lowest time for her. She blamed the menopause but, on reflection, feels that they both could have talked it through and made things work. Her partner was understanding and they communicated well, but Margie also recognised that she needed to get her sex drive back. Now sleeping in different rooms, neither of them had any answers to that. In the end, although they both had a lot of love for each other, the lack of physical contact (not so much as a holding of hands) took its toll and she just couldn't take it anymore.

Feeling as if the relationship made no sense anymore, the act of leaving her partner ripped her heart out at the time, but she now admits she is happy and it was the right thing. Margie states that "If it wasn't for the menopause, I'm sure that we would still be together."

Willing to give love a try again if she meets the right person, today as she speaks, Margie can fully own her menopausal journey. She feels no need to justify her body or manner with anyone anymore. She now feels a sense of freedom on this journey as she embraces the process and shakes off the denial.

Margie admits that she has dated since and has recently ended a two-year relationship with a woman who was younger. Margie doesn't blame menopause this time because she feels they were just on different pages. Margie is still positive that one day she will meet someone with whom she can share her life and eventually get married one day. Fully open to the idea, Margie says, "Bring it on!".

Explaining that she believes that the dynamic of her brain has changed since menopause she now feels more confident, and able to assert herself.

Margie, you came to the interview looking absolutely fabulous. Keep staying true to your authentic self, you are an inspiration.

Sadly, many marriages and relationships do end during menopause but, as with most things, the reasons can be varied.

In a study looking at the impact of menopause on marriage and relationships conducted by Stowe, who are specialist family lawyers and divorce solicitors, 76% of women felt their partner didn't have the knowledge or resources to support them through menopause properly. Furthermore, 68% of divorces involving women at this time of life were initiated by wives.

Menopause is frequently cited as a reason for marriages breaking down. Rachel Roberts, Yorkshire Regional Director of Stowe Family Law, explains, "We are noticing a significant increase in women in their 40s and 50s filing for divorce, citing issues caused by perimenopause as one of the reasons for their marital breakdown. Our study findings supported this view, with 65% of women stating that their perimenopausal or menopausal symptoms affected their marriage/relationship."

(https://www.stowefamilylaw.co.uk/blog/2021/10/18/the-impact-of-the-menopause-on-rel ationships/)

For many, menopause and divorce seem to be synonymous. Whilst it can put a strain on a relationship during this transition period, some couples are able to survive it and remain married. For others, there is a clear link between the onset of menopausal symptoms and the demise of their relationship.

Throughout these diaries, I have tried to ensure that I capture as many different scenarios as best as I can. Quality over quantity. My story is my story and although Nicola, Margie and I have had similar outcomes, there are those relationships that stand the test of time regardless of the challenges menopause can bring. But standing strong, proud and very happy, neither one of us have any regrets as we are ready to live for ourselves, with a new understanding that we cannot control the behaviours of others and a hunger to enjoy our lives the best we can.

I met a lovely lady from India called Tithi. Tithi will be a graceful seventy-four years young on 27th November. Or possibly January, as she explains with a chuckle that in her country birth certificates were not as common. Some people from India are therefore not always sure of their exact date of birth. After a bit of toying back and forth with the two dates, she politely informs me that I can decide. Tithi is one of the few ladies I was unable to video-call. Having never met her in person, listening to her strong, velvety voice leads me to imagine her regal manner.

Coming to England from Amboli, in India, she describes herself as Asian British. Previously working as a primary school teacher teaching ESOL (English as a Second Language) from 1985 to early retirement, Tithi retired following a major car accident when she was fifty-two.

After spending a year off work, she took early retirement when she was fifty-three years old. Not feeling fulfilled, Tithi went back to part-time teaching until she finally retired for good at the age of sixty. At the time of her menopause, she was working part-time and initially, on reflection, doesn't believe that it affected her much. Now in postmenopause, Tithi says that her periods just stopped around the age of fifty-six.

Tithi recognised menopause when it came knocking on her door but wasn't aware of the range of symptoms that she could encounter. All she knew was that she would be hitting a certain age and her periods would be stopping.

Tithi never talked to her doctor, or anybody for that matter, because menopause just isn't talked about in her culture. The same is true for young women going through puberty. Tithi believes that this has changed now with the younger generations, she explains that her daughter, who experienced difficult periods, was able to talk to her and her doctor about this.

During our interview together, we identified that Tithi had experienced thirteen menopausal symptoms. Tithi recalls that many times, she used to make her husband sleep downstairs, having no desire for sex and becoming angry and snappy.

Tithi didn't take HRT or any other remedies at all and just chose to get on with it, often putting her symptoms down to the strains of being busy with work, her house and the family.

As well as her day-to-day stresses Tithi contracted breast cancer in 2016 and subsequently had a mastectomy. Because she had no idea that her symptoms were menopausal and had no idea that there were things you can do to relieve or alleviate symptoms, Tithi just learned to live with it.

Tithi describes herself as an emotional person naturally, so she struggled to differentiate between general daily trials and menopause. Describing herself as feeling emotional on a deep level, she was not scared about what was occurring because she knew that menopause is inevitable for women, so everything that she experienced Tithi put down to being a natural and normal part of the menopause cycle.

With some regret now, she says that if she had known that it was menopause, she would have paid more attention. Tithi recognised she was getting angrier than normal, but again she didn't make any links. Floating between feelings of sadness and then badness, accepting that she had often overreacted, Tithi still couldn't bring herself to apologise to her husband, who would often bear the brunt of her emotional outbursts.

Tithi received no advice from anyone, stating that she never discussed menopause with her husband because she didn't even know herself. Tithi reflects on her life and her marriage and confidently says that she stayed with her husband until he passed away, admitting to having had ups and downs but they stuck together.

"Yes, he often slept on the sofa and I took my anger and frustrations out at him and I never apologised for my actions," she says. "But we stuck together."

A good piece of advice from Tithi to her sisters is, "Try to understand what is happening to you and what you feel so that you can recognise whether it is menopause or just you. Only then can we make the relevant changes."

That is great advice, Tithi, and the Sisterhood thanks you.

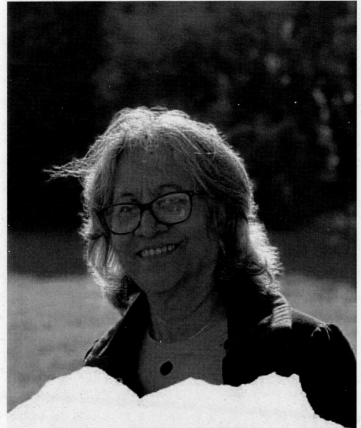

"Seek an understanding of
what is happening to you"

TITHI GHOSH

I don't think there is any one answer as to why some relationships fail and others do not because we are all unique. I believe there can be multiple reasons, from age to experiences and where you are on your own personal journey. Communication is an important part of having any successful relationship and to communicate it must be done properly. We need to talk, listen, and then act on the information we receive because otherwise, it is just a paper exercise. Any form of trauma can cause us to develop behaviours that don't always serve our needs and that can bring further complications too.

As a child, I encountered lots of painful experiences, and now realise that I developed a range of coping strategies to protect myself from further pain.

I recently learned about trauma on a deeper level by studying the works of Dr Gabor Mate. He advocates that all human beings have a true authentic self. He teaches that trauma is the disconnectedness from that true authentic self and healing is the reconnection with it. A very simple but very profound way of looking at trauma and its impact. He teaches that disconnection comes because it is too painful to be ourselves. Trauma is not the bad things that happen to you, but actually the things that happen inside you because of what has happened to you. Examples of this were evident in my responses to my hair trauma experiences.

Sometimes, people come into our life for a reason, sometimes a season, and on the rare occasion, for a lifetime. When we remember this and keep at the forefront of our minds that we are on a journey designed to bring out our best life, we can move forward, learning quicker, feeling deeper and growing stronger.

In other words, let's learn how to be mindful!

Postmenopause

Mindlessness to Mindfulness

I am now in the Big M. I have done my research. I know where I'm at. From excess house clutter and old unworn clothes to my second husband, I've cleared my life of anything that doesn't serve my needs. I'm ready to live my best life. So, what's this all about? Postmenopause? This is the new you, this is the life after all your eggs have finally gone to bed. No more childbearing for us, as we enter this final stage of our hormone cycle. Most of us will either have chosen not to have children, or they will be almost grown, if not already. We should feel refreshed, renewed, excited and proud. Because we made it.

If done right, this is the time when you come to understand all about this natural transition. You have finally realised that you have things that you still wish to pursue, dreams that you want to bring to life.

Do we embrace it? Not initially. Why, you might ask? The main thing that jumps out for me regarding this part of the journey is that, just like waves crashing down on rocks, a current of stress usually takes hold of most of us unexpectedly, affecting our whole life. It can feel like you're drowning and gasping for air without pausing to think about what to do, there just isn't time. So many changes and most are unpleasant. Most of us use the last bit of sanity to try and tread life, while we are trying to figure it out.

It's a big transition and I get that. It's huge. Although it's a natural part of mid-life, what a heck of a ride your body and mind have just taken! So, as with most pain and trauma, we choose to fight or flight.

I remember feeling as though I was in the grieving process. Emotions fluctuating from fear to dread, moving to acceptance, then back to fear, and spiralling downwards as if to my own death. Seriously, at times I truly thought that I was dying. It took a lot to pick myself back up and brush myself down, but I did it.

As I became more aware of the fact I had been living in a mindless state for the last few years, I realised there was a pivotal moment. Before my menopause, my life appeared to be almost perfect. I had a successful business, rental properties, a job that I loved and my children. I had just met (or entangled myself with) my second husband and I thought this would be my forever person.

The more I thought about my whole life journey, the more hours I spent reading self-help book after self-help book, reflecting on myself and my development, fine-tuning every aspect of my life. I suddenly realised that although I genuinely felt happy, I had not reached self-fulfilment at all. I had to remind myself that life is about lifelong learning, even when all seems well. Because no sooner did my life hit that peak of happiness, my menopause started to creep in like a thief in the night. It took hold of my life, and made me question my whole being, bringing that mountain of joy tumbling down.

I had to remember that I was in control of my life, my attitude and my destination. Pondering the beauty and happiness my life once was, I drew courage from within and reminded myself that all things are possible. Although I felt extreme confusion as the symptoms took hold of me, the ones that made me forgetful and feel powerless, I knew I had read enough self-help books in the past that I could centre myself again and I also understood I could breathe in these moments.

Mindfulness, as this practice is known, is when you pay particular attention to all things around you, living life in the moment, not in the past and not in the future. It is grounding yourself. It is not just paying attention but remembering how to pay attention to all things, doing this with kindness and open loving arms when dealing with yourself and others, welcoming each moment with love.

Most people who know me well, usually associate me with the saying, "Kill them with love."

This is a mantra that I use when reminding myself to stay in peace amongst the daily ills of this world. I learned from a young age that the world at times can be a cruel place, but we are only in control of our own actions, and not those of others. Through practice, I realised that if you shower someone with so much love, even if they have bad intentions, it can affect them positively.

I remember to practise an attitude of gratitude every day and remember that I am blessed. Having this attitude has always been a powerful practice in the past and helps to prevent negative energy. People do have ingrained in them a fight or flight mechanism. Another saying of mine is, "The Devil can't stand around angels too long! It makes them uncomfortable."

Anything you repeat grows stronger. We all know this. The more we do anything, the easier it becomes, so be mindful. Be aware of the words that you use when you talk to yourself. Try not to judge others or situations but look at all things with love.

For a moment there, I didn't heed my own advice. I remember thinking I was dying. Joints aching, head hurting and hormones raging, all coming to taunt me after I had endured the trauma of losing my son to Her Majesty. Although he was back now after his 'short vacation', it took me about two years to stop the feelings of anxiety. I had dropped back into daily negative self-talk and felt like my cup was half empty. Scared to allow myself to be happy for fear of another trauma coming to rock my world. I became that person whom I had worked hard to turn away from for most of my adult life.

Ms. Empowerment, a strong and fearless lady, had turned from the lion into the lamb.

However, I caught myself and did a complete one hundred and eighty-degree turn. Here I am now at this very moment, walking away from my second marriage, releasing this incredible man with as much love as I can muster. Although I still love him, I understand that he is not the one for me. I remind myself of all those lessons on my spiritual growth journey that I had already taken the exams for.

The most important lesson: I love myself more.

Becoming mindful and living in mindfulness can be empowering. I have heard this amongst the journeys from many of our sisters. One of the most powerful moments, first and foremost, was the recognition of the changes that they were going through, which led to a new sense of freedom.

So how did I start, you might ask? The most important lesson was acceptance. Accepting who you are, who you used to be and who you may become. Accepting your own mistakes, without judgement, as well as the errors of those around us. Secondly, I believe in nurturing yourself to develop courage and remembering that we are all vulnerable human beings on our own unique journeys. Remembering that we do not own anyone. We cannot force change on others. We can only accept and make the changes for ourselves. I had known of this before, and I had lived in peace. I was ready for this peace again.

I knew I had to accept where I was in my life to allow myself to move forward.

I think my first recognition was my children. I realised that I had spent most of their life striving to be the best mum ever, someone who was as far removed from my own experiences as I could be. As I said in an earlier chapter, sometimes we can hold on to something so tight that we can cause damage without realising it. Well, as I nurtured that small child within me, I realised that I had been searching my whole life to raise my two children without them feeling the things that I had experienced. I realised that, at times, I had gone to extremes that were not always in their best interests.

I thought about what this looked like, and it was the times when I gave them too much materially. This was particularly so with my first child. He became spoiled and I adapted my parenting style when I had my daughter. There are seven years between my two children.

Striving hard not to spoil my daughter, I unfortunately slipped back into this behaviour as she entered her teenage years, particularly when the things that she requested were linked to triggers from my own past. Remember the hairstyles? Well, this is what it looked like. It also looked like over-loving, which can develop into co-dependency. This was something I had to readdress as my children had missed out on vital life skills due to this.

I chose not to be too hard on myself, as I understood that I was not the only woman who had made mistakes with their children. I know that my children have always been my everything, but I had to learn to breathe and allow them enough freedom to make decisions for themselves. I had to accept that they may make mistakes and this was out of my control.

Choosing to stand in my own truth really helped me to stay grounded and start to remember who I was: a powerful woman, with a whole life ahead of me and dreams still needing to be fulfilled.

As I have said, during the interviews, many women confirmed to me that once they had grounded themselves, things became easier. Two such women are Christine and Gillian.

Christine is from the USA, fifty-one years young. Her ethnic make-up is a beautiful blend of Italian, German, Irish and Polish. Happy to be interviewed after our meeting on social media, she loves to share her experience and also learn anything that she might be missing. Christine teaches yoga full time in various locations, including fitness and yoga studios.

Christine is currently in her perimenopause and is living in anticipation of the end of her periods. Some months she describes as quite ugly, the times when she has heavy periods. Starting her symptoms at around forty-five years old, her revelation happened when her gynaecologist mentioned menopause at a routine doctor's visit. Admitting to only knowing that menopause happens when you get old and that things get crazy, this brought a spotlight out on things that were already happening that she had not noticed before.

Christine feels that in America, menopause is not entirely taboo, but it is not talked about very much either. She feels that she had the support of her gynaecologist, who allowed Christine to make choices for herself. She was given lots of advice about what the interventions would do if she chose to go that way. She was also given the option to allow the menopause to progress naturally without any medical interference. The doctor's words were, "We don't want to take your sparkle away!"

Experiencing eighteen symptoms, she only experiences hot flushes occasionally now. Christine recognised that she was gaining weight but feels that her yoga and regular workout routines have helped her gain more muscle and keep any weight gain at bay. Christine has recognised that her night sweats have also eased off along with insomnia and joint pain. She has also cut her hair short to bring its shine back after losing quite a lot during this phase.

Christine laughs when I ask her if she has noticed an increase in irritability? She laughs which seems common for most women and admitted to managing her symptoms with natural remedies, alongside yoga and meditation.

Recognising that if she does not meditate daily, she admits that she would suffer low moods, so she makes this a part of her daily routine and values its benefits. Christine says that the meditation, in particular, helped her with her irritability. Admitting that she also experiences electric shocks, but before today she had never once connected this to menopause.

Christine questions whether she should stop teasing her body with exercise, feeling as though her perimenopause had been going on for so long. "Does my rigorous exercise regime contribute to this," she asks, as she aches for the stop of the flow.

Informing me that her most emotional and scary time was when she had the worst period of her life. She thought that she was literally going to bleed to death. The periods were unmanageable, which then contributed to Christine slipping into a deeper emotional state, spending the time crying all day as the emotions overwhelmed her. Having to take iron tablets due to the huge amount of blood loss, she felt out of control.

The lack of control was the worst, not having the answers to her fears about the situation. Having had a grandma with Alzheimer's, Christine became increasingly worried as she herself began to experience memory loss. Was it her brain's perfectly natural reaction to her being so busy with work, or was it the beginning of something worse?

Admitting there were some funny moments, she remembers looking for her keys once and after a long time trying to leave the house, she couldn't find them. After searching for ages, she finally gave up and went to get some food and found them in the fridge. Now, when she loses her keys, the fridge is the first place that she looks.

Finally, taking hold of her life, Christine started understanding that there are stages to this transition and knew that she had to start to accept this. Fully aware that she is still in the first stage and she would need to make changes to get her all the way through, Christine admits that when she altered her mindset and accepted that nothing will happen on a prescribed timeline, her epiphany came and she found more peace.

It took her a long time to come to this but instead she now tells herself regularly that she is one month down and closer to the end instead of, "Oh my goodness! I have my period again!"

Christine is a firm advocate for surrendering and says she has been preaching this for about a year now because this is when she started to feel more empowered, strongly believing that her meditation and yoga have been the biggest help in accepting and surrendering to the process.

Christine says, "Even if you don't feel as though meditation is your thing because you don't think you can keep still or quiet your mind, still give it a try! Give yourself at least two minutes a day, find a quiet place and just breathe. The body is still going to do whatever it wants, so be kind to it and just allow it to do what it needs to do. Relaxation comes when you start to breathe and the stress levels will come down."

Gillian, another stranger to me, is also a yoga instructor, whom I was introduced to through a friend. Originally from my hometown of Leeds in the UK, she now lives in the city of York where I went to college. Within her work environment, Gillian feels that menopause is talked about within her world but what she hears from others in relation to medical support is, in her opinion, atrocious. She believes that a lot of women appear to be struggling, mainly because of the lack of support from doctors and others being unable to manage menopause professionally.

Forty-four was the start of her perimenopause, and now at forty-nine years old, she has been working through her menopause, as a self-employed yoga teacher. Gillian has done menopause training in the past and in the near future would like to put that to use in a more meaningful way.

Currently in perimenopause, she was unaware of the exact stage that she was in. Symptoms started to become recognisable around the age of forty-four when she noticed that her period cycle started to become irregular. Gillian recognised quite quickly that she was entering this transition. Due to the previous training through her work and spending time around groups of women who had shared their experiences in different workshops, Christine feels lucky to have been able to share their experiences. At the time she remembers being horrified and scared at some of what she heard.

Gillian also had a range of symptoms that she had not associated with menopause. Still today, she feels that although she felt some symptoms quite badly in the beginning, they were easily managed after being put in touch with a homeopath. Within days, symptoms were managed and her remedy was tweaked later when the symptoms started to come back. In total, the remedy has been tweaked about eleven times, but it has worked to suppress the symptoms every time.

Gillian admits to responding quickly and making big changes to her diet at the start, which she feels had a positive impact on her digestion and weight gain. She says that the changes she made have been drastic, so this has improved things quickly. She no longer eats bread or drinks alcohol because these sorts of food were creating sensitivities that caused a lot of discomfort. She has also chosen to only go down the natural remedy route, recently purchasing some herbal remedies.

Gillian has experienced a range of emotions and feels that she has, "a lot less tolerance and patience for most sh*t!"

She has become angrier, and at times feels scared about her health, confessing to having a nightmare only the previous night, questioning whether she will stay healthy enough to be around for her son. Being a single mum of a twelve-year-old, she feels it's vital that she is okay and this can often prey on her mind.

When asked if Gillian is finding some humour in her day to day, she tells me that she is. Just the other day whilst doing some online shopping, she said she felt a bit more relaxed and cared less about social norms. Being given the opportunity to choose her title, she rebelled against being called Miss, Mrs or Ms, she happened to scroll down further until she noticed that the other options were Dame or Lady, so she opted to be a Dame for the day which made her feel good.

In some senses, Gillian feels like some things are less of an issue now, confirming she is more passive about life and often cares less. "But in a good way," she tells me, jokingly, going on to explain that in other ways, she cares more. The emotional changes have increased her confidence, meaning less cowering and being much more likely to stick up for herself instead.

Yoga, therapy and training have been positive and she is also well trained in the line of being a womb yoga teacher. Gillian feels that all the experience and education she has around women's issues have led her towards a positive experience with her own menopause.

She now manages her diary differently, keeping more time clear for herself each day; whether that be for gardening, window-shopping, having a coffee or just having more time to sleep. Doing all this to reduce her stress levels, a penny only dropped recently when someone said to her that she shouldn't be making these changes just for menopause. Instead, she should be doing these things for herself anyway. Now she priorities herself and looks after herself everyday. Gillian feels sad that it took her so long to work this out.

"Our perception of menopause as a society is so negative that it makes me sad," Gillian says as she goes on to tell me about her studies of the moon and how the moon has a connection to a woman's menstrual cycle. Feeling sad that menstruation wisdom is not known by the masses, she describes menopause as a stage of life where there is the potential to feel like a Queen. It makes her sad when she hears about the lack of recognition from the medics, a lack of wisdom and respect for this stage in life.

She feels that women's bodies have been messed up and doesn't believe that medical professionals give women enough choice before offering them hormone-altering treatments. Gillian says that even the contraceptive pill and coils can allegedly affect a woman's menopause but doesn't think women are taught this. There is no knowledge or education from the people who prescribe these things and no open dialogue at all.

Our potential for wisdom is stripped from us by society. Although she feels positive about her own transition, she also recognises that it is quite early in her transition and is aware that her symptoms could become worse or unmanageable.

Sometimes people want to know how you gauge that something has been a success. How do we get to a tranquil state of peace? I believe it is different for everyone. Christine found peace in a change of attitude, Gillian found peace in finding time for herself and the small daily pleasures.

The penny also dropped for me this year, when my daughter got her first tattoo. On her right thigh, it was a lion's face. She smiled as she informed me that it reminded her of me!

"Remember how you always say "put your lion face on"? Well, I want to be able to always look down and be reminded of you!"

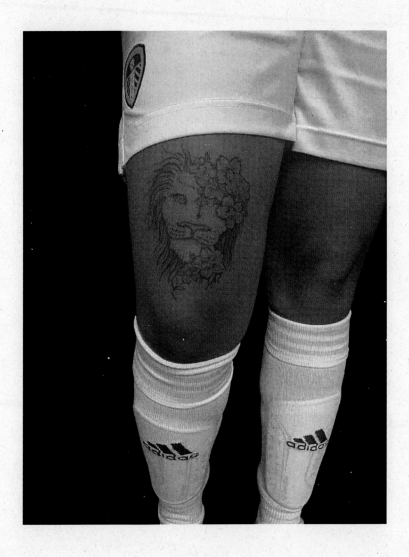

With all this being said, my menopause and I will continue on this path and into the next adventure. We will be patient with each other and kind. We will be there for each other no matter what the future holds. So how do you do that? You need to find what works for you and that can present itself in various ways. Let's have a look at what solutions life has on offer!

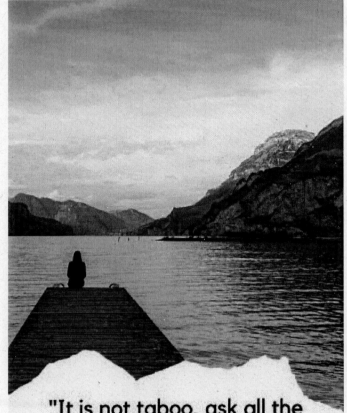

"It is not taboo, ask all the questions and find all your answers"

CHRISTINA DECILLO

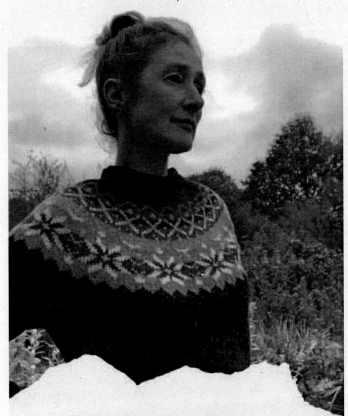

"Centre yourself and get
support"

GILLIAN SHIPPEY

Nature, Nurture or HRT...

Is it in the stars, your tea or some other shit?

It is 2020. In America, Donald Trump is fighting for power for a second time, Britain is going through the Brexit shenanigans...yes STILL! I was also told recently that I'm ending a seven-year cycle. Not only a seven-year cycle but a seven-years-of-bad-luck cycle, so I quickly reflect on the last seven years for insights. What have I experienced? It is only in the previous seven years that I have been with my second husband. We got together in 2014 and got married in 2016. Yes, a fair few uncomfortable, annoying and tragic things have happened since.

My menopause also started two years ago (possibly before that, but at least two). Then we have the Black Lives Matter movement over every channel on the television at a time when menopause hits and you are generally at your most emotional. When you are a black woman and you see this onslaught of police brutality, it is a tough one. Tough to watch and tough to accept that this is the society that we still live in. Also, on the internet, we observe the extreme weather cycles linked to climate change. The world can be a very scary place.

This makes me reflect on all the growth and all the healing work that I have done on myself over the years, only to be reminded that we still live in a very broken and cruel world. Emotionally, it affects you, and for some women menopause heightens their feelings so much that they cannot help but allow the emotions to be all consuming.

Recently, I was at a wedding talking to a friend of a friend, then out of the blue, I began to engage in some deep and meaningful conversations about the seven-year cycle. I happened to mention that, for the last year, I had been highly addicted to burning lemongrass in my diffuser. Thinking it was because of the beautiful aroma that pulled me in, I was swiftly informed about the poignancy of this practice.

Unknown to me, lemongrass in all its forms, is brilliant for the mind, body and soul and is even considered to be something close to magic. With strong anti-depressant properties, lemongrass can help you to overcome misery and improve your mood whilst repelling negativity from your home and warding off evil. It is also said to encourage lust and promote honesty within relationships. Drinking dried lemongrass tea is also said to improve psychic abilities. Burning lemongrass can help to remove or overcome obstacles in your life to help you let go of, or move through, difficult situations. I was informed that the lemongrass scent is my body's way of choosing to say goodbye. I thought deeply about this and it made sense. Even on a subconscious level, I guess we can say goodbye to things that no longer serve us.

I am a Gemini and although I do not read horoscopes from a magazine anymore to find out how my day is going to pan out, I do think that when I read the character traits of astrological signs there is a certain accuracy to the description of me and other people I know. Inquisitive is my middle name and I love to try new things. I love to learn about all the different things that interest us as human beings. Recently, I have been intrigued by the concept of quantum entanglement as introduced to me by my brother. I love anything that gets me in touch with connecting to different energy vibes.

I am a positive person so, regarding my menopause, I was thinking that if I'm optimistic, grounded and have a good support network, and still feel as though it is the worst thing in the world, how do those women who are not as confident as I am and do not have a good support network cope?

I have met women who swear on the benefits of meditation. Not that I am a guru or anything, but I meditate at least a couple of times a week because there are definite benefits in learning to regularly relax your body and your mind. I can see why women seek out alternative therapy because menopause can be so brutal.

From speaking to my beautiful queens, one thing I know is that menopause implants a certain confidence and fearlessness into even the quietest and timid of people, but how do we get to that point? I know that we must take matters into our own hands and try to find what works. Let us meet some of the other ladies and see what they have tried.

When speaking to the queens, I met Sara. Sara is currently in perimenopause and is forty-three years young. Sara had confirmation ten months ago but believes she had noticeable symptoms approximately nine months before this. Although she found it really tough in the beginning, she has come to terms with it and manages it well.

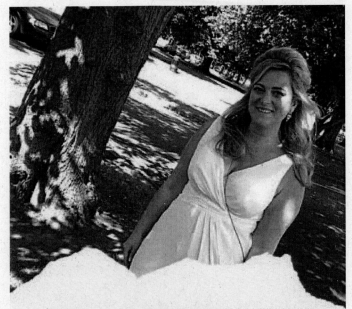

"Pain is something we have to embrace and learn to breathe through. Embrace the change. Embrace the growth. Your body has got this!"

SARA MEEKLEY

Sara is a woman who constantly measures the lunar cycle and how it impacts her symptoms. This is the first time that I have seen somebody do this, although I am sure there are thousands of others out there. As I sit listening to Sara, I cannot help but admire the amount of detail and time that goes into her day, plotting the position of the moon against every feeling and wave of emotion she endures. I genuinely found it unique and fascinating reflecting on this practice. Although I will never have the time nor the patience, I can clearly see its benefits.

Speaking to Sara made me think about the diverse ways that women seek or find in order to cope with such a trying time in our lives. For Sara, this was not a brand-new concept as she has often used this practice throughout her womanhood to plan her period cycle. She found that it really helped her menopause symptoms to use lunar planning regularly. Sara realized that after the first four months of tracking her cycle, she could clearly pinpoint the times when she was performing at her best. More importantly, she was able to identify times when she may need to be much gentler with herself. This meant that she was able to plan her tasks wisely, leaving any important meetings to other days if the moon was not looking like it was in her favour. She says it helped her to understand so she did not panic as her body faced a wave of changes at this time.

Having a word with herself, at a pivotal moment, Sara reminded herself that she was entering her golden stage of life and that she could take this journey wherever it may lead, determined to try to enjoy this stage as best she can. A supportive boss told Sara that she will feel more in control when she gets her head around it. It was the fear of not knowing what was happening that propelled Sara to use the planning to ensure that she could be forewarned and thus forearmed.

Using the planning meant that she was aware when she may potentially have more sleepless nights or when she may feel more anxious and she is now able to make time to be on her own when required.

Experiencing eighteen identifiable symptoms during this transition, Sara decided that she did not want to take HRT. Trying a few different herbal remedies, Sara confesses that she finds using a more natural angle and plotting her cycles on the lunar calendar to be the most beneficial. When asked if she would recommend anything else she recommended the natural remedy, sage.

Still in the first stage of her transition, the perimenopause, Sara has things under control. Finding out that she had entered menopause only came when her supportive manager at work pointed it out.

"She runs the department I am in," Sara says. "She was my lifeline."

It was reassuring for an older woman to support her and point her in the right direction, offering suggestions or different solutions and reassuring Sara that what she was feeling, although bad, was quite normal.

Sara's first thought was that it could not be menopause because what she had heard about was not as bad as what she was experiencing. Her symptoms were so awful that she was ready to call an ambulance. With a playful giggle, she tells me that she remembers asking her manager what she was going to do now, pointing out that they worked in an office full of men. Sara recounts fondly how her boss got a book and photocopied relevant pages, handing them all out to the staff to let them know how they should be supporting Sara and her other colleagues on this journey.

Choosing to tune in to the natural rhythms of her body, Sara was convinced that there must be some logic behind the body choosing this new phase. She felt as though she had entered a natural grieving process, with the body holding onto its last set of eggs. As the body is designed to procreate, she feels that the overwhelming emotions that women feel are the body's way of grieving when the eggs are not inseminated each month. It is about letting go of a part of her life where she is not going to make any more babies. Hearing Sara make sense of this aspect of the process made me more mindful about it.

Sara goes on to say that if it was not for her colleague at work and the sisterly humour they shared, then she does not know how she would have done it. She jokingly describes the menopause as, "totally ridiculous, init?"

She goes on to say, "I have to laugh, otherwise I would cry, because there are times that you felt quite scared. And I do not have any contact with my family, so the sisterhood was important."

Thank you, Sara. I am so happy that you have found the right strategies to help you make sense of the pain. I am sure a lot of your new sisters will find this useful as they recruit you into your new family, your global sisterhood. Welcome, our sister, welcome.

Let us meet Rehana. Rehana's 'go to' was a natural approach. Transitioning into early onset menopause at thirty-five years old when her mum sadly died. At the same time, symptoms of M.E (Myalgic Encephalomyelitis) had started making it difficult to differentiate between the two. Recalling a memory of lying on the floor at her job on several occasions because she remembers just being so exhausted that she couldn't move.

At the time, Rehana did not know what was happening. She is unable at this point to remember if she had hot flushes as she struggled with memory loss due to a benign brain tumour a couple of years before. Not taking HRT and preferring to support herself with natural remedies, she also had a friend who was a nutritionist and helped Rehana through her transition. This is her story.

Currently sixty-one years young, born in Pakistan, she moved to Glasgow aged three and now lives in London. Mostly retired apart from some volunteering for Age UK supporting people with Dementia, Rehana's previous career was challenging. She worked as a social worker throughout the duration of her menopause.

Rehana starts by telling me that, culturally, girls were brought up to believe that periods were something to hide or be quiet about. Watching her mother go through menopause from a young age, she remembers her experiencing awful symptoms.

All of her sisters started menopause young, also in their forties. Rehana started even earlier than that, aged thirty-five. Questioning if it is genetic, she also remembers her mother having a hysterectomy due to her severe symptoms and luckily it sorted her symptoms out. Before this, even though Rehana was young, she remembers watching her mother practically banging her head against a wall whilst having an episode. It did not stop there as both her sisters struggled with menopause too.

Feeling a little guilty, Rehana says that she struggles to remember her own symptoms, but this may be due to the lasting effects of the tumour. Within her culture there have been improvements in how open people are now compared to when she was young. Her family are more traditional than some Pakistani families and her mother came from a generation where she just didn't talk about periods and menopause, maybe out of a sense of shame. However, she informs me, that it is not the case anymore for lots of families she knows.

"I don't really speak to my sisters much about the topic in detail and that is a generational thing," she says. "But young people are different. They are much more willing to talk."

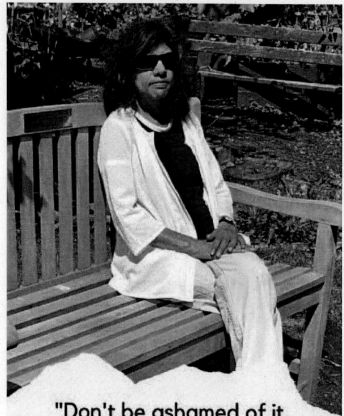

"Don't be ashamed of it.
Be open and willing to talk
about it"

REHANA MALIK

Although initially, Rehana did not link her symptoms to menopause, on further reflection she was able to identify quite a few. It is hard to think that after identifying at least eighteen recognisable menopause symptoms, Rehana endured this without her sisters' support, not having any friends who she could share these feelings with. One saving grace was that Rehana was in a long-term relationship with her husband, who was very supportive and never made her feel embarrassed. She knew she could talk to him. Rehana said he was very open and honest: "We were very close."

When Rehana was thirty-five years old, her mum sadly died and her periods just stopped. Around this time Rehana also found out she had ME and she believes the onset of this was connected to her mother's passing, believing that her body somehow went into shock. Everything became, in her words, "topsy turvy."

Due to the trauma, she went into early menopause, enduring her perimenopause for a few years. Following this transition, osteoporosis also set in quickly, but Rehana believes this was inevitable after having rickets at a young age and already being vitamin D deficient. "Once bone density decreases, you cannot reverse that, but you can keep it at bay," she says, as she describes what she has done to keep herself healthy.

Choosing to nurture herself, Rehana's natural remedies included a much better diet and vitamins and minerals like increased magnesium. Rehana had a blood test taken and was sent to a biochemist and was told what vitamins and minerals she needed. Rehana says that this made a huge difference to how she felt. Reminiscing about being referred to a biochemist and nutritionist many years before in 1987 and over time they became friends. They are still friends today.

Her least favourite stage was perimenopause as that was when her symptoms were fiercer. She periodically became distressed because she felt overwhelmed and out of control of her emotions, saying she could burst into tears at any moment of the day and the smallest thing could send her into an emotional state. Although also struggling with memory loss and having a mind that went blank, leaving her unable to keep up with the flow of conversations, Rehana admits the scariest time was having to lie on the floor in the office

"I couldn't even sit in the chair; I was so tired." She smiles now as she recalls thinking, "I hope no one walks in."

Being unable to control her body was frightening.

There were some funny things she recalls: "I was once in a meeting and got very red-cheeked looking like I had blushed and people thought I was embarrassed about something that was said but I was hot and sweating and did not know what to do. I wanted to run out of the room, but I could not leave the meeting, so I just had to keep going."

A few years in and Rehana had a poignant moment where she had been feeling quite stressed and had woken up one morning and it just hit her. This thing was happening and it was what it was so there was no need to worry about it or get stressed about it. She says it was a bit of a light bulb moment. Thinking only positive thoughts and focussing on the blessings, one of which was not having any more periods because, as Rehana informs me, she had hated them so much. She was also excited about the sexual freedom that came with that.

Never having had children due to contracting blood cancer when she herself was a child, Rehana recalls that she had always wanted them but never could. Sadly, she says, "I'll never quite accept that decision life had for me and some days I can deal with it better than others. I know I'm more accepting of it now than back then, but children were something that I wanted".

Being supported by an amazing nutritionist friend who told her right from the start that they could sort it, and that she would be fine and not to worry, Rehana felt good and was able to be honest with her, "woman to woman". She says, "This helped because I went into menopause earlier than a lot of my friends so they couldn't offer advice, but were still very supportive."

Still positive, Rehana confesses, "I struggle to separate my menopause from my mother's awful experiences. When I remember mine, I automatically remember my mother's. I was very fortunate that I was in an age and era where it was treated and recognised differently from when my mother went through menopause back in the sixties. A sense of 'thank goodness' but also very sad for her and what she went through as it was horrendous, and witnessing it as her children, it was very hard. Attitudes to menopause in the sixties and seventies were not great. Now it is a bit better and hopefully the future is even brighter."

Sara takes an approach that is linked to nature and Rehana takes a more nurturing approach, so what is all the talk about HRT? Several women I interviewed had taken HRT with varying degrees of success. I admitted to our next lady during the interview that I had never wished to take HRT due to the negative press associated with taking this drug. Subsequently, since starting this project, I have learned much more about it and realised that HRT is considered one of the most effective solutions for the relief of menopause symptoms despite concerns over the potential risks to aspects of women's health.

In the early 2000s, after the published results of a study suggested that extended use of HRT may increase the risk of breast cancer and may increase the risk of heart disease, panic amongst some users was created and the overall use of HRT dropped by around sixty-six per cent. Since then, the use of HRT has been safely restricted so that only the lowest effective dose is prescribed. For many women using HRT for short term treatment, the benefits outweigh the risks. With the correct dose, duration and regular assessments from your GP, HRT can be a life-changer.

One woman who openly discussed taking HRT was Sally, who at fifty-one years young, is white British, born in Newcastle upon Tyne and currently living in Leeds.

Sally is currently in perimenopause and has started taking HRT, following a recent programme on television, which made her aware for the first time that it was more beneficial to start HRT earlier rather than later, if you are going to take it at all. The decision was not made to manage symptoms but replace the depleted oestrogen levels that she now faced.

Sally has been using a type of oestrogen supplement for a while now following a routine smear test in which she was told she had a thinning vaginal wall. At the time, she was unaware if this was age or menopause-related although Sally explains that she knew it could be.

Some new symptoms started fiercely at the beginning of the year, which led Sally to assume that she was moving into menopause and having an older sister who was experiencing severe symptoms already, Sally describes thinking of this as, "the awful menopause stage."

She contended with bouts of anxiety, night sweats, hot flushes, and insomnia. Initially, Sally didn't put all of these down to menopause and the words she used to describe the feelings at the time were, "feeling like a failure in all areas."

I discussed this with Sally, informing her that lots of women feel this exact same way. The symptoms passed quickly. Unable to get an appointment to see her GP at the time, she says that, on reflection, if she could have seen the doctor, the brief symptoms she experienced were so bad that she would have started taking HRT there and then. Today she reasons that because symptoms were fleeting, it could be down to the general stresses of everyday life.

Informing me that although her mum doesn't talk about menopause, she has a very good dialogue with her sister, which has led Sally to feel like she is one of the lucky ones. Her sister experienced excruciating symptoms which initially caused Sally to dread even the thought of menopause. Sally is happy to have someone to communicate with and feels fortunate that she has not endured the same fate as her sister, when she describes the photographs her sister shares regularly of her nightwear soaked in sweat.

Although Sally's mum is anti-HRT, she still chose to try this method, describing her attitude as wanting to live life the best she can: "I want to live, while I'm alive."

As well as her mum, Sally feels that societal perceptions are "rubbish". Describing herself as a "trailblazer", because as an older mum, Sally describes herself as a very open person who has offered support to lots of friends around the subject.

Sally has looked into the risks and explains the social pressure she can sometimes feel as she explains that because she had her children at a much older age than her current peer group, there is a certain pressure that is felt when her peers are going out and drinking. Understanding that these are the sorts of behaviours that could lead to a higher breast cancer risk whilst taking HRT, Sally chooses to live a more modest life. Not wanting to make taking HRT a higher risk due to drinking too much, Sally is happy with her choices but doesn't feel as though society sees this as an acceptable excuse.

One day, prior to taking the HRT medication, one of Sally's sons asked her what she had been buying. Looking confused, she realised that her son thought that she had been shopping and she was looking at a long receipt. In fact, she was reading the comprehensive instructions from the HRT packet. The instructions and possible side effects information was huge.

"But in fairness," she says, "This would be the Same for a packet of paracetamol. You must research and make sure that your information is up to date. It is important to look at your lifestyle and eliminate anything that may put you at more risk."

A dog walker by trade, Sally also feels that her active lifestyle helps her to stay healthy and feel better.

Sally says that in some senses she feels "a little bit fraudulent" when questioning whether she took HRT a little bit prematurely. The depletion of oestrogen helped cement her decision because, at the time that she started to take it, which was only two weeks previous, she was not experiencing that many symptoms. One experience which was new is lethargy as she reinforces the difficulties in knowing which symptoms are menopause and which are generally old age.

Overall, Sally experienced seventeen symptoms and was visibly shocked at the revelation that electric shocks were also a symptom of menopause. Sally admits that she still has difficulty knowing what is and what is not menopause.

Like many of us, she experiences bouts of brain fog, where she will forget what she has gone into a room for or opening a cupboard and not remembering why, she has to sometimes talk to herself and, "have a word" as she strives to stay positive and think of her cup as half full.

Sally feels that she has a really great doctor and feels very lucky. Aware that not everyone has the same experience, she feels it is an outrage that GPs don't have to go through any specific training around menopause. After all her research, Sally also admits that she was not one to take medication previously, but she feels that as long as you do your research thoroughly and weigh up the pros and the cons you should be able to make an informed decision about any medication and take it if the benefits outweigh the negatives.

Sally ends the interview by warmly informing me that she feels that although men won't ever be able to truly appreciate what a woman goes through, she has made both her sons aware of menopause. By explaining what she is going through to them, she gives them an understanding but also ensures that they are prepared for the future.

Thank you Sally, it was a pleasure to meet you and we welcome you as part of our Sisterhood.

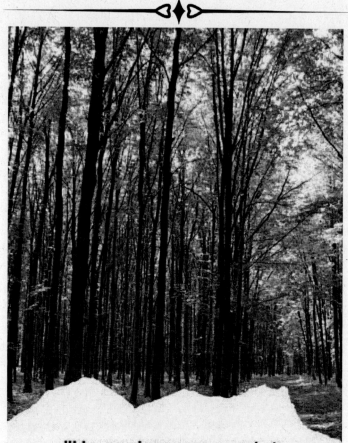

"Up to date research is key"

SALLY CORK

Well, what's best? Nature, nurture, or HRT? I think it should be a personal choice. Having spoken to several women, I can see clearly that what works for one does not necessarily work for another. Find what works for you and do your research. Talk to people and do not be fobbed off by your GP or other medical professionals. Keep asking until you find the answers and try things to find that old vibrant you again. Write things down. This usually helps with our brain fog anyway. It helps to keep a diary of your symptoms so that you can reflect and notice if things are working and if they're not you can make and track changes more effectively. Please do not take everything at face value, take advice from your friends and family, but always remember that everyone is individual and unique.

I have faith in you, my sisters. Once you find the right combination, it should not be hard work, but it has got to be the right combination of remedies for you.

Speaking of work, this might be where other fireworks start to fly! Shall we take a look?

The New CEO:

'Certified Extinction of Ovulation'

Most of us spend a third of our lifetime at work, so it is only fitting that we look specifically at work and how this may impact our current existence. It's okay me asking you to be mindful about how you treat yourself but what about others and the way they treat you? The actions of others can hinder our growth, so let's look at one of those areas where we may need more support. One of my favourite authors has this saying in one of her books: "When you see crazy coming towards you, just cross the road!"

But what if you can't cross that road because the crazy is in your job, disguised as a vindictive supervisor or co-worker. Worse still, what if the crazy is you?

I guess it all starts with education. After finishing my time at school, one of the main things I remember was the excitement in the air as hundreds of children started talking about their futures, questioning where they were going after their exams, what they were going to do and ultimately, what they were going to be! I never particularly 'liked' school and after spending years being told that I wouldn't amount to anything, I learned quickly that only I could be responsible for my own destiny.

Real school wasn't nurturing to me. Bullied at home and being fed negative dialogues at school, I learned to be my own advocate. I think this is what led me to develop an aura that some people found hard to deal with. I know over time, some people have made many negative observations about me, such as, "Look at her with her big car, who does she think she is?"

I really don't care what people think and people will always talk. I know that if I could re-enact a scene from the movie Scrooge and call it instead "The Ghost of Childhood's Past" most people I know would never wish parts of my childhood on anyone.

Secondly, if people spent a week shadowing me, when I was setting up my business and really saw the hours and hard work I put in, most wouldn't want that either. People never really know what a person has been through to get to where they are in life, and there was a time when I just wouldn't care about their opinions. These days I can ignore it and hope they will show more empathy towards others, one day. I will always support people to reach their goals, as I know it's not easy. After my childhood experiences, I remember another school I went to that had excellent facilities: it was 'The School of Hard Knocks'.

I realised that the best place to learn about things was life itself. I started to look at my whole life as a university. I realised that life would teach me better things and there would be exams too. Some I would pass with flying colours and others I would fail. There were always chances for re-sits and I would get out what I put in. I told myself that the best thing to do to get ahead in this world was to be a strong advocate and be diligent.

"Give your best in any job that you do," I would tell myself. "And if you can't climb the ladder, build your own!"

There is no relevance in my first few jobs delivering newspapers, in fact, no relevance at all for the first ten years of my career. The sad thing is, when discussion about menopause did become relevant, whether it was to assist me to be a better colleague and support my peers or when the big M loomed in my own future, it still wasn't there. I don't ever remember, not even once, in any of my jobs (and I have had a fair few) anyone telling me even an inkling about what would one day transpire. Therefore I was never destined to be the best employer or colleague because I was never given the tools.

In 2019, when I started to have my first inkling of my new friend Big M, I owned my own company and I immediately began to investigate how to perform better as a supportive employer. I initially started my business in 2010, and embarrassingly, I must admit that I had never given menopause any thought at all.

With the new hints that this may be my next chapter, I researched online and started implementing policies that supported my employees and myself. As I researched, I became even more aware of the many different symptoms. It further cemented my inclinations, as I read the horror stories of what a woman's body can endure, and I realised that I was already in this living nightmare.

Granted, my GP had still not confirmed this idea, but I felt intelligent enough to draw my own conclusions with the help of Doctor Google. Regardless of my lack of attendance at medical school, I started to notice symptoms in my employees that I felt were probably connected to this phase. I implemented a 'Menopause Policy' that outlined some of the symptoms so that employees could better support their colleagues experiencing menopause and feel that I did all the right things, ensuring that every employee read the company's new expectations. I also became an even more sympathetic boss in my approach to staff who may have been struggling. I must admit that I did feel guilty for not knowing about it before.

Recognising the signs and having to endure the constant memory loss, I was scared about the foreseeable issues this may cause with my work. Like clockwork, my spirit started to talk to me. She whispered lovingly in my ear, "Get a PA and this will be the answer to all your concerns."

As I questioned the voices, asking important questions about how I could justify what seemed like a luxury and affordability, my spirit held me steadfastly and as usual, let me know that all would be okay. Like most times when I put my trust and faith at the forefront of my decisions and ride the positive energy waves, it all worked out.

A few weeks later the name of a young lady, whom I knew, popped into my mind. My spirit said this young lady would be perfect for the job. I hadn't seen her for ages due to the government lockdowns, but lo and behold a few weeks later and completely out of the blue, she cheerfully informed me that she was visiting soon.

When she came to visit, it was a beautiful sunny day. After a bit of a catch up and a walk around my new beautiful zen garden, I told her my thoughts and that big signature smile appeared. She gleefully informed me that the timing couldn't have been more perfect as she had been pondering a change too.

After working her four weeks' notice and starting a journey together, we have been getting on like a house on fire ever since. I have the peace of mind to know that any important business won't be forgotten and she is learning lots of new things. Don't get me wrong, my memory is actually not as bad as it was in the beginning because I think your hormones eventually level out over time. This means that sometimes, I'm happily reminding her of things too!

In all my years as an employee and the ten years in my own business as an employer, I hadn't heard a whisper of this strange new affliction. Not a word within work but even more worryingly, it was like pulling teeth trying to get an open dialogue with the people who vowed to do no harm...GPs! Most women I spoke to had negative experiences when trying to discuss our new friend. Annoyed at this observation, I started to look at the world holistically to try to see if this was the case everywhere.

Speaking to our queens, ninety per cent of them didn't get much in the way of support, if at all! Speaking to friends, both male and female, it was also around ninety per cent of them who confirmed that it was indeed a taboo subject where they lived.

Aging is viewed very differently across the world with some cultures believing that people of a certain age should be respected and celebrated, while in others, old age is often presented negatively.

In western cultures especially, there seems to be a shared attitude towards aging and it is associated with immobility and an inability to work. Care homes operate as a common destination for the elderly in western cultures. In contrast to that, most Asian, Mediterranean and Latin American cultures usually have elderly family members living with younger family members in a large household and are typically well cared for.

This is a little similar for menopausal women - in western patriarchal cultures, older women seem to be viewed as less valuable members of society but this isn't a common attitude throughout some other cultures, who believe that menopause can be a profoundly useful and spiritual time in our lives, representing the transformation from the old self into the most powerful versions of ourselves.

When you think of all the opportunities that we miss for educating and arming our children, it can be frustrating. I spent many a day educating mine and still made plenty of mistakes, but when I knew better, I did better; not just for my daughter but my son as well. I'm sure my future daughter-in-law will thank me one day.

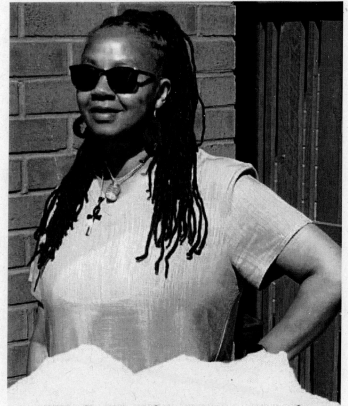

"Embrace the process and
don't be afraid"

PHYLLIS WOODLY

To get some perspectives other than my own, I spoke to Phyllis (an employee at a school) and Sara (a manager of a large team of mostly men but with a few menopausal women in the mix). Both ladies have different experiences to share.

Phyllis sits in front of me in a regal manner, a huge smile painted across her face as she eagerly awaits the looming line of questioning. Phyllis is fifty-two years young, the only one of her siblings born in the UK. All her brothers and sisters were born in Saint Kitts and her mum travelled to England while pregnant with Phyllis. Describing her family as black Caribbean, she also informs me that her grandfather is mixed race. Her maternal grandfather came from Portugal and settled in Saint Kitts and her dad's side of the family came from San Domingo in the Dominican Republic, also settling in Saint Kitts.

Phyllis is unaware of exactly how long she has been in her menopause but thinks it is roughly three years. Describing it as something that just came out of the blue and, smiling, she told me that people at work would inform her that she had gone a bit red. Phyllis says that she never hid her new condition and would let her colleagues know what she was experiencing, trying to get them to take her condition seriously.

Further explaining how menopause affected her, Phyllis says that when her symptoms came out of the blue, she started with flushes that hit her physically in all parts of her body, which resulted in feeling anxious and panicky, unaware of how to control them and what to do.

After several bouts of these new symptoms, she made the link as she had friends and sisters who were already experiencing menopause. Phyllis laughs at the irony of her preconceptions as being "merely a stage when women can enjoy not having periods anymore" and "just getting a bit warm."

Unable to gauge what stage she was in at this point due to a hysterectomy, which resulted in her periods stopping, she did speak to her doctor however. She was swiftly informed at the appointment that she was probably in menopause, so no test was needed. HRT was offered as a solution, but Phyllis declined.

Although Phyllis experienced nineteen identifiable symptoms such as joint pain, hair loss and weight gain, she did not want to take HRT, guided by her elders in her community. The elders informed Phyllis that HRT was not good for her so she instead opted to try herbal remedies, the main one being sage tea. She also tried to eat healthy food but admits to still eating sweets from time to time.

Feeling as if, for the most part, she has it under control, Phyllis says there is no pattern or a decline in symptoms. Although admitting that at times symptoms can just disappear, she said they will still return just as fiercely. She says she is at the stage now where she knows what she's dealing with. Never feeling scared,

Phyliss says she still "doesn't like it one bit; but it is part of the natural cycle of a woman" so it doesn't scare her. She doesn't let it run her life, which she sees as being about living and embracing. As she says this, her beaming smile appears again.

Having lost a child many years ago, Phyllis now has two sons. She chuckles as she informs me that they laugh at her from time to time, when she forgets what she is talking about mid-conversation.

"The kids are good. They know Mum's going through menopause," she says playfully.

Discussions were initiated by Phyllis to help her sons understand what she was going through. Explaining why she was extremely tired and at times overwhelmed is what prompted Phyllis to speak to her children. She says they have been very supportive and understanding and subsequently, they help more around the home too.

Employed as a teaching assistant, Phyllis explains that she does cover as a HLTA (Higher Learning Teaching Assistant). Informing me that she has worked all the way through her menopause, I ask Phyllis about her experiences.

At Phyllis's work, they organised a wellbeing committee which was initially put together for the well-being of the staff. Phyllis's input was raising awareness around menopause and facilitating ideas on how to support the staff. In Phyllis's employment, there are a few women who are currently going through menopause.

Some of the ideas brought forward involved equipment such as classroom fans because the classrooms are warm. This followed a few incidents where Phyllis felt like she had to actually get up and leave the classroom as the heat seared through her body, giving herself time to get herself back together.

Unfortunately, nothing materialised from those meetings. The old headteacher left and meetings have resumed again with a new headteacher. Fans were brought up in a meeting recently and she is hoping that things will improve. Phyllis advocated for the women and boldly told everyone that unless you are going through menopause, you will never fully understand it, informing them that it is a serious subject and not something to take lightly.

Explaining to the participants that, unlike other illnesses where people may take time off work, sleepless nights can be a regular occurrence of menopause and teachers are then expected to come to work and teach without any support. The feelings of anxiety can affect how teachers or employees in general perform. Having a new female boss, whom she believes is yet to experience menopause, Phyllis realises that she may not be able to have the full empathy of a boss until they themselves have endured it. She observes that for some of her colleagues, her workplace may not feel like an environment that all women would feel comfortable in to discuss menopause, even though Phyllis and a few others are.

Another request was for some tangible policies to be written that support the staff. Phyllis says there is currently nothing in place. Although recognising that there are times when she has had a bad night's sleep and she could do with a few extra hours in bed, she states that she wants to be all about living; always trying to embrace it, she remains upbeat and positive, striving to live her life in a positive manner.

When she is mindful and catches herself in the moment, she allows herself to be still, reflect and embrace her menopause, thus allowing herself to recharge and get her energies back.

Phyllis ended her interview by saying that she thinks that menopause needs to be highlighted and recognised as a natural part of a woman's journey and that menopause is an umbrella term for the symptoms because everyone's journey is different. Although she is not looking for her eighteen-year-old self again, she is looking to be healthy and describes the process as enlightening for her to understand that nothing is to be taken for granted.

Support groups and other platforms need to be in place so that women do not see it as taboo. However, it remains taboo. Phyllis wishes that there were more forums out there for both women and men to understand and she reaffirms that policies need to be in all workplaces to ensure that women are supported.

Still learning about life and herself, she says "menopause is not nice, but there are also other things in life that are not nice too, so we need to try to embrace it and stay grounded." Her final note was admitting that she is still learning.

Thank you, Phyllis, for being a strong voice for others. Your sisters thank you too.

Sara G is the supportive boss whom we heard about in Chapter Ten. She starts her interview by fully owning her story and agreeing to use her real name.

"I'm not precious," she says, as we discuss the various bits of housekeeping. Settling in to start, I couldn't help but share a snippet of the positive things that her employee had said about her as an employer and how the impact of her acts had affected her employee profoundly.

Currently fifty-one years young, Sara is from Leeds. Of mixed heritage, her dad was Spanish and her mum is from the UK. Managing a telemarketing team, Sara is Vice President (VP) of Market Engagement for the business. She has worked throughout her menopause and was recently promoted from Head of Market Engagement to VP.

Previously experiencing anxiety due to other life challenges, such as divorce and being a single parent, Sara was fully aware of what anxiety felt like. This time, it was different and the anxiety manifested itself in anger and tears.

Experiencing eighteen symptoms, Sara recalls observing her mum going into menopause. Her mum suddenly became "dithery" and totally lost her confidence overnight and it never came back. This meant that Sara had these perceptions in her head.

Sara explains, "When you understand it and can put a label on it, then it's better. You are frightened for everyone around you. If people knew you before but then you suddenly turn into a different person, it makes you start to question what is going on here." She continues, "Once you understand it and can share the information with your loved ones, or even colleagues at work, everyone can settle in with an understanding, giving those around you the tools to be able to handle what is going on better."

Feeling as if the whole process was hard, Sara describes her day-to-day struggles and doesn't feel as though she got support herself, even though we already know that she was a support to her employees. When she transitioned from perimenopause to menopause, it was during the government lockdown of 2020. Experiencing emotional effects, Sara laughs as she recalls that due to her work position she struggled and found herself going off to try and regularly compose herself, then coming back and apologising for whatever debris she had left behind.

"The attitude at work," she says, "Is to just crack on. You have got to.".

At home, Sara explains that because she is very open when communicating about her menopause, she gets support from both her partner and her daughter. Feeling like she wears a variety of hats at home, they know when Sara is not in a good place and leave her to enjoy her own space. However, she says that in the beginning, it wasn't always the case.

As she describes the beginning of her symptoms telling me the impact it had on her personal life, she explained that she had reached a point in her life where everything was perfect. She had just met a new partner, bought her dream home and was in a great job that she loved. It all sounded very familiar to me as she explained that suddenly the anxiety set in. Experiencing mood swings, she started to get angry and was picking arguments irrationally and overthinking things. She explains the dialogue in her head as "almost narcissistic" because part of her brain was reasoning with her and asking her what she was doing, while the other part was totally unforgiving.

Sara describes herself as not generally emotional, preferring to go away into her own room and cry on her own, not liking people to see her. Sara informs me that there were many times that she cried, often for things that were very small incidents. An emotional experience that happened recently, which mortified her, was when Sara was in a meeting with the company Managing Director (MD), the chairman and the company Chief Executive Officer (CEO). Getting angry in the meeting, Sara proceeded to cry hysterically, blubbering when she was trying to talk and unable to stop. Although the situation eventually worked out in her favour, Sara feels that responses from men can be quite patronising. Sara describes the meeting as highly emotional, unprofessional and that she felt like she was out of control. Sara received apologies from the "big wigs" and it wasn't long after that when she was offered the promotion. Positive benefits resulted but she was still mortified.

Feeling lucky that she was informed by her doctor a few years ago that she was entering perimenopause, Sara says she is aware that for most women, this support is not there. Life became easier for Sara as she was able to understand the transition better.

It was at the point when her doctor recognised her menopause that Sara started to feel better. Previously she was blaming herself for these uncontrollable behaviours but now she knew it wasn't her fault. She was able to put it down to her hormones and not feel as though madness was setting in or that she was being generally unreasonable to those around her.

Having a best friend who has also joined Sara on this journey is helping her to keep "in the loop" along the way. Chuckling as she recalls the interaction on the day, Sara's friend bought her a book which is what she used to distribute information to her team to support her menopausal ladies.

Choosing to ensure that she keeps an open dialogue with those around her, Sara will clearly inform people when she is having a moment and explains to them that she will come and chat to them after.

Sara says the response from her male employees has been great. In a team of around fifty, with eighty per cent being young males, Sara feels that they accepted the information gracefully.

Facilitating the understanding within her team, she distributed information to support others to know how to communicate better with the ladies going through the Big M. She made sure that they also knew that it was something that could benefit them outside of work, as most people will be in contact with other females too.

Sara thinks the younger generation is possibly better at understanding what is happening than people from older generations. Sara feels that the company benefits from pro-actively supporting her employees to be aware of menopause and not see it as taboo, as it helps the employees to understand and not take things personally, thus contributing to a happier environment in the office.

"Awareness is important," she says.

Sara feels that there are lots of myths and she wants the perceptions to be challenged as she feels it is currently seen that women going through menopause are old and unable to be funky and cool. Proudly she informs me, "This is just not the case."

So that's work from a few different perspectives and what I found to be beautiful is that our sister Sara was the boss of one of my other ladies. The positive impact that Sara's supportive approach had on her sister employee was worth the effort.

Dear Sara, thank you for being a trailblazer for the women in your team. We hope that many people take a leaf from your book. Your sisters are lucky to have an amazing boss like you.

Not getting all statistical, but on a general note, I have heard that many women leave work or change jobs around this age and I can hazard a bet that it's probably due to issues that could be resolved with a bit of support.

The media is only recently making menopause a more regular topic of discussion, but I feel that we still need to do better. Where does it start? I feel it should start at home. Employees are our children but "all grown up."

We nurture them and get them ready for school and then the school should continue with this trend. It hasn't happened and it has never been the case, but let's start today. If I give some tips in the next chapter, will you promise? Let's walk together then.

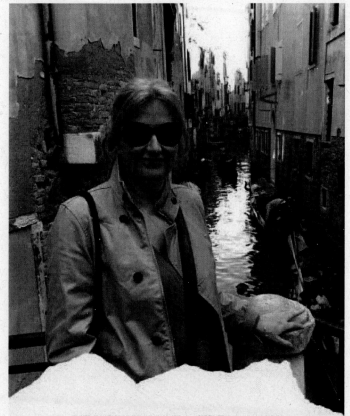

"Embrace it...this gets easier"

SARA GILMARTIN

Coming Full Circle...

Daughters become Mothers and Mothers become Daughters

I decided to get a bit of fresh air with you guys, so here I am at the side of the pitch, watching my daughter play football. I can see Charlie up ahead. I hope she's got my coffee. I'm thinking about a few things today. This is my daughter's last season before she finishes college. She currently plays for Leeds United Under 21s. Next year, she wants to go to America for four years of university on a football scholarship. It's been a goal of hers for the last two years. As she excitedly plans her future, I remember those days; the dreamy days. Thinking about your future and getting excited as you sample the experiences life has to offer. So, I've been trying to plan for this move and help her to achieve her dream.

Funnily enough, it makes me think of a time I went off on a trip to the other side of the world. Full of youthful curiosity and a thirst to learn more about my culture, I met a man whom I started dating when I was around eighteen. I left my dad behind in pursuit of this stranger, whom I had been writing letters to with pen and paper...do you remember those days? The plan was to go and stay with him on the nature island of Dominica for six months.

Looking back, I must have broken my dad's heart. My kids only need to go as far as the corner shop and I think about them, wondering if they are okay when they are gone for more than the ten minutes it should take. I can't imagine what was going through his head (or mine) at the time. Admittedly, I only made it to the three-month mark because I missed home and the other boyfriend whom I had left behind in England. Please don't judge. It only happened once, but I soon learned juggling any more than one man was tiring, to say the least.

Looking back, I had an amazing experience. This is where I learned the most about my hair. I became friends with a lady who was a hairdresser. I would spend hours in her salon and experiment with various styles. I went to my first basketball game and listened to so much live music because the man I dated was in a band. This is where my love for reggae music was born. Obviously, I had heard reggae music before and was quite fond of it, but there is something magical about live music that touches different parts of your soul.

With my daughter thinking about her future, I was reminded that menopause is the time we can often reflect on our motherhood. We torture ourselves at the thought of them flying the nest and over-analyse any effects our behaviours might have had on them, wondering what the future holds. I love my children so profoundly, but I don't own them. They are only on loan to us for a short time. Our job is to try our best to teach them the skills needed to live their own lives; support them to find their purpose and, in the process, love and care for them the best we can.

I believe I have often over-loved my children. They know it and I know it, and we have often talked about it. I think that is, sadly, a symptom of my own shattered childhood, never wanting them to experience the pain and trauma that I went through.

I am glad that I over-loved them instead of under loving them, but holding onto anything too tightly can still break it. So yes, this chapter is about parenting, and obviously it's about parenting in menopause too. We already know that my children had a word with me when I wasn't looking after myself. We know that my son and I often spend quite a lot of time together and my daughter has her beloved football. My own childhood has affected my parenting and I think this is the case for most of us. I am not saying it always has to be negative, but our experiences do shape our future behaviour. During the years when I should have been nurtured as a small child, I was forced to grow up too quickly, often taking on the adult role in the house when my mum made unsafe or irrational choices.

As part of the process, I found it beneficial to regress and reflect on all areas of my life as I wrote this book. I believe strongly that there are things that can affect us even though we would never think about it on a conscious level. Regressing means that you can go right back and clear any lingering issues, transparently looking at any trauma to see where it needs healing in order to move forward.

Within my periods of regression, the things that weren't explained to me as a child would cause me pain and I would often have to work things out myself. There is a reason that children are not allowed to make certain decisions until a certain age and it is because the mind is not considered mature enough. Here I was, raising myself and trying to figure it all out. As well as not having the relevant guidance, I also didn't have consistent love and security. Many things happened during the tender years of my childhood that I won't elaborate on too much here, but it should be noted that the most significant part and the ending came when my mum allowed my stepdad to throw me out of the house when I was just thirteen years old.

I stayed in a few places and when my dad finally found out, I moved back in with him. However, during my periods of regressing, I now saw the devastation caused by such rejection from my mum. I was able to own the truth of this situation and realise that the over-loving of my children came from the constant under-loving I had endured. I was able to forgive myself and the little girl inside me. She had concluded that I had to hold onto my children so tightly so that they would never have to endure this kind of pain.

I addressed the guilty feelings that arose when, even though I felt I gave my children lots of love and guidance, my son still went on to make that poor decision which resulted in him being taken away from me. It prompted me to think about my son and the direction his life went in when he explained to me the missing piece in his own life: a father who had never shown him 'the man stuff'.

Things like learning how to shave and what it takes to be a man. Even though I thought I was doing a good job, the lack of the right male role model had a profound negative impact on his development.

The process started and it was deep. I had to do the work. Luckily, I did the work with the loving support of my children, who listened to me reflect and shared their own pains. Together, we worked it all out.

Motherhood has a profound influence on our children so I think it's important that we own our experiences and think about the impact they might have.

That's a bit of my story. Now let's meet some of our ladies. Meet Averil, Barbra and Jayne. All mothers with different parenting experiences. One thing I noticed from each and every one of them was that they all had a shared experience of being the strong ones. Neither reaching out for help nor allowing themselves permission to make mistakes, they moved forward with an acceptance that this is just life.

Averil is sixty-seven years young, originally from Scotland and now living in Leeds. At the time of her entrance into perimenopause, Averil worked alongside her ex-partner, running a business and had a part-time job in a pub. She was also a mother of six children, informing me that she had worked since the age of fifteen. She currently works in payroll but informs me that she has done lots of different jobs throughout her career to provide for her family.

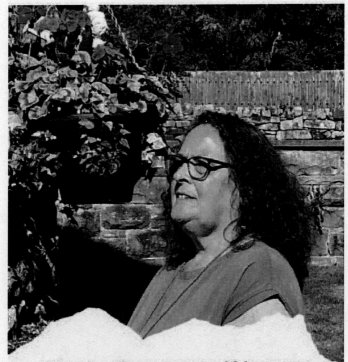

"Look after yourself better.
Without good physical
health, you can't have
good mental health"

AVERIL MACGILLIVRAY

Unaware of the different stages, Averil tells me that her menopause is long gone. Averil said that there was no significant time where she stopped and identified what she was going through because she says she was just too busy.

Finally, Averil did stop and reflected upon the fact she hadn't had a period in a while. At the time, for a brief moment, she thought that she might be pregnant. Having a history of irregular periods, Averil also experienced getting pregnant whilst taking contraceptive pills. There was no regular timeline she could measure anything by. She realised that she had gone through menopause and, as far as she was concerned, it had been quite painless; certainly nothing like the horror stories she had heard about.

Although Averil thought she had experienced menopause unscathed, we identified during the course of our discussion that Averil had still experienced nine different symptoms. These included hot flushes, weight gain and low mood.

At the time, she took evening primrose oil after someone suggested it; but Averil didn't really notice it making any difference. No longer experiencing any symptoms, Averil recalls that the mild symptoms suddenly stopped at some point but says that they were short-lived and hadn't left any impact mentally or emotionally.

As a mother, Averil used to get really stressed about money whilst raising her children. She doesn't think that her anxieties were anything to do with menopause.

"I'm generally quite tough. I don't give into illness easily," she says. She then chuckles, "I just got on with it. When you have so many children, it's just what you do."

Averil talked about the monthly cycles with her household and laughs as she recalls how manic it was having four daughters in the house, all menstruating at the same time. "All lined up and all bleeding at the same time because of the moon cycle", Averil began noticing the hormonal clashes and thinks that's why she embraced the end of hers.

In later years, when discussing menopause with her children, she recalls with a chuckle that she informed them that she didn't really experience any behavioural changes: "One day, having a girly day on Mother's Day, I told the kids I was never moody and denied any knowledge of experiencing anything. All four daughters spat their drinks out in unison as they couldn't hold back the laughter."

They confirmed to Averil that she had been "an absolute nightmare" and "a bad-tempered old bag" as she put it. The kids felt Mum's irritable reactions were more common and her fuse was definitely a bit shorter.

On reflection now, and since that day, Averil admits at the time that she had a son who was going through 'a naughty phase' and another son who was socially isolated. Other ongoing emotional issues with one of her daughters and her own personal life led her to believe that any mood swings were simply a justifiable reaction to what was going on.

Averil has recently started having an open dialogue with her children and is confident to speak to them about it, chuckling as she informs me that she has been honest and sends them to Doctor Google when she doesn't know the answer to their questions.

Averil recalls the advice given to her by an old work colleague, who said that long walks really helped her. Heeding this advice, Averil has found real benefit in taking walks through the countryside. She also makes sure that she drinks plenty of water. Leaving us with some positive advice of her own, Averil says, "Look after yourself better and look after yourself more. Do the groundwork before you get older because physical health is so important."

Shall we move on and meet Barbara?

Barbara is another lady who has emigrated to Bulgaria. At fifty-three years young and originally from Hampshire in the UK, Barbara owns a bar and hotel, where she is the head chef.

Right off the bat, Barbara informs me that she thinks her interview will be boring because she didn't really experience anything, although admitting she has a friend who is currently going through loads. I remind Barbara that every woman's journey is unique and of equal value.

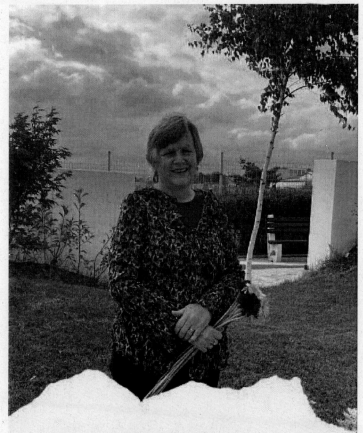

"Don't worry about it and it
will be okay"

BARBARA BURCHELL

Postmenopause for the last five years, as a young lady she always had irregular periods, so is unable to accurately pinpoint when she actually started.

Barbara is not aware of when she went through her perimenopause. Working as a hairdresser at the time and after having the Norplant implant, (a contraceptive implant that lasts five years) Barbara went on to develop ovarian cysts. The cysts burst and she was rushed into hospital to have an operation to treat these cysts. Barbara then began to experience several issues with her periods including them becoming irregular.

At the interview, we identified that Barbara did have some symptoms, but up to now has never associated any of them with her menopause. She did experience weight gain which she has now got under control.

Never taking medication such as HRT or any other remedies, Barbara admits that she just got on with her life, recounting that she only really thought about it before she went into menopause. She worried that she might get some bad symptoms after her friends told her plenty of "horror stories" about menopause.

Barbara feels that societal perceptions are not good and that society doesn't talk about menopause enough, even though it is a part of life for all women. She adds that her own mum never spoke to her about it. A point of reflection for Barbara as she admits that she hasn't spoken to her children about menopause either. She has two sons, one daughter and a granddaughter. Informing me that she didn't have any symptoms and neither did her mum, she also assumes that her daughter will also follow this trend. This is her wish. We can only hope, for the sake of her daughter, that this wish comes true.

Starting our next interview, when asked if she is ok, Jayne tells me that there are "a few trials", but she is coping and is just taking each day as it comes.

As we settle in, Jayne informs me that she is a qualified chartered accountant and owns her own accounting company. She tells me that she might not be that far into her menopausal journey so she "might not know that much". Unable to identify the stages, we establish through our discussion that she is in perimenopause.

Jayne is fifty-four years young. Born in Harrogate, Jayne moved to Leeds as a child and has been here ever since.

The first signs that she noticed were lighter periods, but has not had any tests to establish her transition. Noticing that she has got quite weepy lately and unable to identify the cause, she adds that hot flushes have recently started as well. We established that she has nine recognisable menopause symptoms.

Jayne, like some of the other women, had put them down to other things (work, children and everyday life). Jayne admits that the doctor has put her low moods and brain fog down to stress. Not having had a period for approximately eight months, it took her about four or five months to notice this. Lately, she has been getting her words muddled up and this seems to be increasing. Jayne informs me that her kids find this hilarious. It's a strange feeling, she says as she describes the steps she takes to jog her memory. It seems like Jayne is familiar with the brain fog too.

Jayne's prior knowledge of menopause was that periods stopped and you started to have hot flushes, but that was where her knowledge ended. In relation to societal perceptions, Jayne says, "Like a lot of things, it's not talked about."

Noticing that with each generation the communication gets better, Jayne still confesses that she has yet to discuss this stage with her children.

Having one daughter and one son and being close to them both, Jayne feels that menopause may come up in conversation at some point, but she recognises that her daughter experiences heavy periods herself, so she does not want to burden her with her own issues.

Happy that she is now more informed about what other changes her body may endure, she laughs as she tells me that she will look out for all the symptoms that I have mentioned.

Jayne explained that she has always been an emotional person, but the difference now is that she can burst into tears and she doesn't know why. Recently, while out on a walk at the reservoir with her son and the dog who had run on ahead. Jayne suddenly stopped, sat on a bench and started to cry without any apparent reason. Eventually, coming to find out where she was, Jayne recalls the dog being concerned about her emotional state, her son being more accustomed to Jayne's tearful ways.

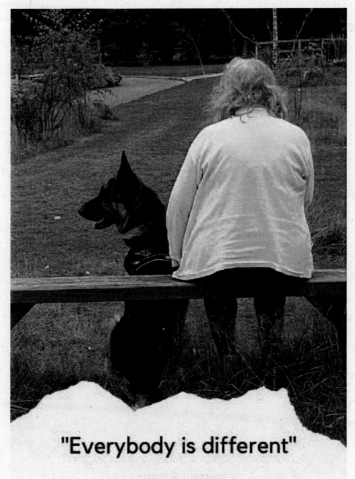

"Everybody is different"

JAYNE PICK

The scariest thing for Jayne at the moment is that she doesn't feel in control and doesn't feel as though she knows enough about menopause. Going to the doctors at some point is one option, but at the moment, there is a lack of desire to do that because she feels they are "too busy, have enough on their plate and don't have time for such trivial things". A common theme?

With the final question, when asked about her children's understanding of menopause, Jayne confesses that she has been on medication for stress since shortly after her symptoms had started and her children are aware of that.

At this point, Jayne cries as she considers the impact that her menopause may be having on her children. Through her tears, she expresses concern that her son may have noticed a difference in her over the last few months. Unsure if her daughter has noticed anything because she lives away at university, Jayne admits that they don't talk about menopause.

Jayne apologises for becoming emotional and I tell her there is nothing to apologise for; I reassure her that hers is a vulnerability I recognize so well. We are all women, and we all go through this transition. Looking like she has the weight of the world on her shoulders, she explains that she has had quite a bad week at home. Her son, who has been struggling due to his own ill health, can also pull on her emotionally.

Agreeing to some 'me time' she then composes herself and says in true Northern form, "It's the Yorkshire way. I'll be reet."

What does this chapter tell us then?

My first thought is that parenting is a minefield. However, the beautiful realisation is that we are all connected and that, for mothers, there is a special connection to our daughters. It has nothing to do with favouritism. I always thought that my son and I had a closer relationship than the one with my daughter because we spend so much time together; I hope that throughout this you understand how truly close my son and I are.

The truth is that my daughter has been forever watching me. I'm her role model, watching every inch of what I do, how I do it, and building her own self-worth. So be mindful, no matter how close we are to them, children usually aspire to the parent of the same sex, looking to build their identity and finding their own true self.

I have learned not to be afraid to regress and reflect on my past. There is the small child in you which needs nurturing. Your daughter's small child needs that nurturing too. There is you as you are now, how you were and who you will become; the same is true for all daughters.

Talk to your children because communication is key. Take time to learn about yourselves. Prepare your children because their journey will not necessarily be the same as yours.

Our daughters need nurturing because they will be a future version of us. Know that we all come full circle. Daughters become mothers and mothers become daughters.

The Real Awakening

"Embrace your old crone"

I know that this journey has caused me to reflect in many ways, but with this emotional labour of love has come so much more growth and healing.

Throughout the book, I have unpacked some private areas of my life to share a journey of discovery, sharing information about my childhood, my children, and love.

It wasn't just about romantic love, it was about love in all its natural forms; the relationship between me and my friends, my son and daughter, my family, romantic love and my connection with the world in general. Reflecting on pain brought healing and allowed me valuable space. Regressing to my prior self and transgressing the menopausal taboo, I have now learnt to live mindfully in the present.

In this chapter, you will meet my last two queens, Carol and Fiona. Both sisters whose emotional crossing into menopause touched me deeply. Both spoke fearlessly about their transitions' impact on their mental health.

Carol tuned in to the interview via video link from the beautiful island of Dominica, a mountainous Caribbean island with natural hot springs and tropical rain forests. At fifty-eight years young, this beautiful lady moved back to Dominica two and a half years ago.

Originally born in Bradford in the UK, she moved to Dominica during her childhood then returned to the UK for a number of years before finally heading back. Although born in the UK, Carol sees Dominica as her home.

As we sit down to talk, Carol laughs nervously as she wonders what might come out of her mouth and muses over the choice of having a pseudonym. Deciding to take the leap and truly own her own story, she informs me to go ahead and use her real name.

Carol was unaware what stage of menopause she was in but, after a bit of discussion, we were able to pinpoint events and it was clear that she is now in postmenopause. Carol is a freelance artist by trade and was working as a tutor for Leeds Mind (a local mental health service) during her perimenopause stage.

She was in her late forties when she started to experience anxiety and mood swings. Although she admits it was not very clear, there are still pivotal landmarks she is able to recount in detail. At the time, not sure what was really going on, with periods that had become sporadic, Carol remembers her last period being around the age of fifty.

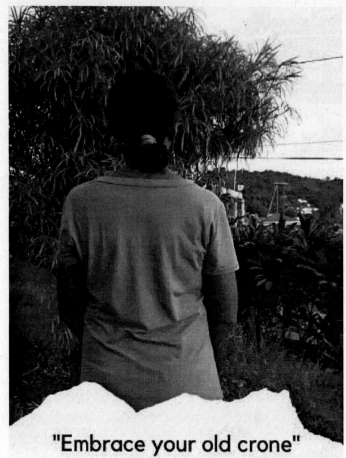

"Embrace your old crone"

CAROL SORHAINDO

Shortly after her periods became irregular, Carol found out she was pregnant. Having miscarried twice in her late forties, Carol tried to come to terms with the prospect of motherhood. Admitting that children had never been high on her agenda, she laughs playfully as she reflects on the stereotypical artist wanting to be creative and free. She did begin to look forward to becoming a mother, but alas it was not meant to be. Carol had another miscarriage. In spite of her initial doubts about motherhood, Carol nevertheless grieved the loss of the child her body and spirit had nurtured, albeit for a short time.

Shortly after this, her doctor informed Carol that she had no more eggs. Carol found herself grieving this second loss, trying to come to terms with the fact that she would never again have the chance to become a biological mother.

Pondering the different emotions, Carol recognises that she was happy when her periods stopped because it brought a real sense of freedom.

Her hot flashes introduced themselves just before her fiftieth birthday. She confesses that the symptoms she started to experience at this time had to take a back seat. As Carol was spending more time in Dominica and planning for her upcoming migration, she was also going through trials such as a break up so she didn't link the hot flushes to menopause.

"Dominica is hot," she says playfully, "So I don't think I noticed them in that warm climate."

Over time, experiencing fourteen recognisable symptoms, Carol only took natural remedies in the form of wild yam capsules. This was following her own research and she says they worked quite well. Unfortunately, the company stopped producing the capsules and she was unable to find an alternative. Making changes to her overall diet also helped and now that she is in postmenopause, Carol tells me that she no longer experiences any symptoms at all.

Going through stages that were very tearful, she believes that some of these were related to reflecting on her current life, her past life, her relationships and other situations. Wanting to lock herself away and not spend time around other people, Carol felt that she was crying all the time.

"Finding it hard to express yourself to people can be quite difficult when you don't have the words to describe what's going on," she says. At the time, she was unaware that these waves of emotions were happening due to menopause.

The high levels of anxiety were a scary time for Carol and she once felt as if she was almost on the edge of a breakdown. Once, when she was at work, she walked in and could not even recognise the people that she was working with. Luckily, she was not very busy that day and was able to take herself off and find her own space. It made Carol reflect on her own mental health and think about how finely balanced mental health really is. Luckily, she was able to get support from both her colleagues and her clients at the time. She reflects that it feels even more poignant talking about it today.

In Dominica, she has never heard anybody publicly speak about menopause; she finds people quite closed about the issue. In England, by comparison, she at least heard a few things about it.

Totally switching how she thinks today, Carol now confesses that she puts herself first at all times. She used to feel guilty because she was always taught to put others first. Even though people are sometimes not happy with this, this is the approach that she has taken.

"Value yourself," she says, "Say no to people sometimes."

Carol says that, at the time of realising she was in menopause, she read a really powerful book that helped her understand her transition. She felt that one of the most powerful messages that she came across was the term, "Embrace your old Crone".

Nobody she knew ever talked about menopause but, as Carol began to open up, so did they. Carol has subsequently recommended the book to various people.

"It's the most empowering thing that women can do, to read about a woman's place in society," she says. "Read about that role and embrace your old Crone."

She fondly recounts the helpful advice she received from the book: "In history, there is the thing about the wise old woman going into the forest and retreating, seeing herself as a wrinkled old thing." But Carol says, "It's a symbol of embracing your wisdom as a woman of age. The wrinkles and the grey hair. It is a sign of change. Embrace the wisdom and all that comes with it!"

"It is a time for women to connect with their femininity, reflect on life and spend time with themselves," Carol says. She feels that the body is telling you that you need a break. "It is like it is trying to tell you to spend time with yourself and embrace the freedom that this chapter of your life brings."

Carol has wanted to move back to Dominica for many, many years and believes that maybe because she was not true to her dream, she was not always fully present in her relationships. Having had two long term relationships in the last twenty years, she says, "It is hard to separate what are real-life problems and what is menopause. Each partner comes with their own stuff too."

Standing proud, Carol has no regrets. She values all her life experiences and says the time was right when each experience came.

When asked if there is any new love on the horizon, Carol says "never say never, but not at the moment. I'm focusing on myself now. It's Carol time, and time for my mum and my sister."

Carol is enjoying being in that space as she describes it as a space of freedom.

I really appreciate the open and transparent account Carol gave me and I believe that these conversations can really help women to open up and find themselves. Thank you so much for sharing, my sister, and continue to enjoy your newfound freedom.

Now shall we meet Fiona? Equally strong, standing with her own truth, Fiona talks to me about her own struggles with mental health and speaks to me with the strong voice that, as women, we all need.

As Fiona sat in front of me, I could initially see the hesitation in her face. Unsure what this encounter would bring, she willingly sits for my line of questioning.

Before starting the interview, Fiona updated me on general day-to-day life. We had talked for almost an hour over coffee before we got down to business.

As with everything in life, everything happens for a reason and that conversation was just the thing to prompt her to relax and warm up, but I wasn't prepared for the overwhelming emotions that were about to spill out.

Fiona is my neighbour; we have lived next door to each other for eleven years. At fifty-three years young, for the first time I hear that she is a beautiful mix of British and Australian heritage. Born in Papua New Guinea, to missionary parents, she came to live in the UK at the age of four.

As an educational consultant, mentor, and writer, Fiona is currently postmenopause but feels as though she is still in the middle of it all. Her symptoms originally started in her mid-forties. She is experiencing nineteen symptoms that are affecting her day-to-day.

At the age of fifty, Fiona got breast cancer. Sadly, in the same year, her dad also passed away. Lack of sleep, combined with her grieving and menopausal symptoms made her feel as though she was going off the rails. Exhaustion had taken a hold on her.

Suffering really badly with her periods, she initially sought advice from the doctor. She doesn't feel as though she received much support. Fiona suggested to the doctor that the cause of her heavy periods could be menopause but, after several visits and referrals to specialists, it was still not recognised. Fiona feels that there is a real blurring of mental and physical health by professionals who do not seem to make the relevant links.

Feeling at her lowest, the doctor informed Fiona that she was unable to take HRT because of her previous breast cancer and she was offered anti-depressants or counselling as her only two options. Fiona chose the counselling, which she took up and paid for privately as she was only offered six sessions with a long waiting list.

During counselling, Fiona was able to explore the emotions that she was experiencing, realising that everything was connected to her grief. Losing her parents four years apart, looking after her father (who suffered with Alzheimer's), having emergency surgery due to pancreatitis, followed the year after with breast cancer, the menopause symptoms and lack of sleep all blurred into one. All this whilst caring for her three young children, the youngest of which was only three when Fiona's mother died. She continued to spiral as she felt her life unravelling right before her eyes.

Fiona didn't have just one scary moment, she had a few. She wept as she recalled identifying her breast cancer, recalling the emotions and the fear she felt for her children. It was an immensely frightening time. Looking like she had the world on her shoulders, it was emotional to watch this beautiful queen as she tried to make sense of this awful experience. I felt as though she was crying for a lot more than breast cancer alone.

Moving on, she tells me that during this period, she was carrying so much responsibility: her children, family, parents, siblings, and students. A powerful feeling came over her at the time, of wanting a space that was just for her, to escape and get away from it all.

Gradually, after the counselling started, she was able to reflect and make improvements. Now sleeping again, she is able to function better. Fiona feels as though menopause gives women a powerful voice and the ability to be truer to themselves.

Observing that doctors separate mental illness from physical illness, she says, "It's not mental illness, it is just lack of sleep. Of course, a year of no sleep will take its toll on you!"

Besides professionals not handling menopause well, Fiona perceives menopause as something that society, in general, doesn't talk about. She regrets never talking to her mum about menopause. Feeling there are clear links between mental health and menopausal symptoms, Fiona observed this with her own mum's experience. Unfortunately, through a lack of communication, it is something Fiona was only able to highlight after the fact, with little to no understanding at the time.

Having a child quite late at age forty-two can in itself impact your energy levels. Admitting that it is hard to know when one issue starts and another one stops, as she said, she regrets not talking to her mum. She has these words to share with you:

Fiona says that "although I don't have a daughter, if I did, I would always advocate talking. Talking to each other and helping prepare the way will help you to break free from any cycles, empowering you with a better understanding and helping you find peace."

Interviewing Fiona is where I believe the term sisterhood was cemented for me. I realised that I had been living next door to this beautiful lady for so long, a lady who was going through her own pain and struggles. I know she wasn't on her own, having a supportive husband, three beautiful sons and close friends, but she was without a strong woman's energy. Women's energy is a powerful thing, and we all need it.

I know myself that when I see certain powerful sisters in the community, my soul sometimes aches for a hug. When I am blessed to share an embrace with my empresses, I walk away feeling stronger, more balanced and empowered.

Realising that we were two kindred spirits going through our own pain and battles, missing the opportunity to offer each other support and embrace our own feminine energy, I wondered where we had become disconnected. I thought about our journey up to now. I realised that, years before, Fiona had offered to pick up my daughter from school. My daughter was around ten years old at the time.

Fiona came home and had forgotten her and, subconsciously, I realised that I had disconnected myself from her then. I searched my soul and realised that, due to my own childhood trauma, I was unable to truly forgive Fiona at the time. I had chosen to bury this in my subconscious mind and told myself I would never allow this to happen again. My daughter was fine, no harm was done, but the underlying fear caused me to put my barriers up.

To Fiona, my sister, I am sorry. Today, I understand that we are all human, and we are all going through our own pain and trials. Sometimes we experience traumas so deep they affect our natural conscious mind. I stand in my own truth today as I say to you, I love you, I forgive you and you are beautiful.

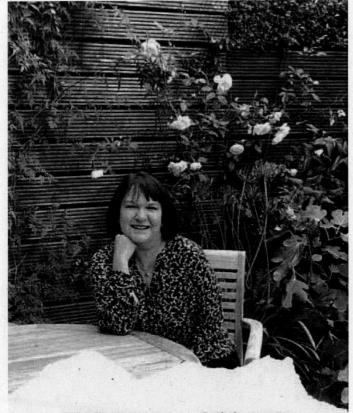

"Talk to your children to
help prepare the way"

FIONA MAIDA

Many women shed tears during my interviews, for different reasons at different times and for different lengths. Tears that signified trauma, pain, forgiveness, triumph, confusion, understanding, fear and love.

So what have I truly realised whilst writing these diaries?

The real awakening is embracing your natural life cycles and "embracing your old crone".

I am not religious, being more comfortable describing myself as spiritual. I read about paganism once and, although I am not a pagan, in relation to women and menopause they seem to have a very good way of looking at this stage in life. As confirmed by Carol, they advocate that we should all embrace our old crone.

The Japanese word for menopause is 'konenki' and generally Japanese women don't worry much about menopause at all. Arguably, this is something to do with the breakdown of the word konenki: 'Ko' meaning "renewal and regeneration," 'nen' meaning "year" or "years," and 'ki' meaning "season" or "energy."

In some indigenous cultures, post-menopausal women have considerable power and status. Menopause is seen as the transition to becoming a spiritual elder. Some indigenous cultures even believe that a woman must enter menopause to access their healing powers because menstrual blood has the power to create life in the womb, so when women reach the age of retaining their "wise blood," they transition into "wise womanhood" by keeping their wise blood within. At this stage in life, women become priestesses and healers — the spiritual leaders of their communities.

Here in the West, women mostly don't regard menopause as a period of wisdom, regeneration, or renewal, but instead it is regarded as something dreadful that will eventually happen to us; something that we have no control over whatsoever.

Menopause, years ago, used to be called 'the change' and women 'had to go through the change'.

'The change' is about the only thing I remember my mum ever telling me about menopause. In this hush hush society, all cloak and dagger, there is a silent revolution brewing.

If done right, women can enter this stage empowered, fearless and excited. But it takes a village, and that village means all of us. As women, we must first take ownership of our own attitudes concerning menopause. Change the dialogue, both within ourselves and to each other. Someone said whilst being interviewed, "how can we expect men to understand, when we don't even understand this stage ourselves?" There is a lot of truth in that statement, so I am hoping that, as Queens, we take a stand and embrace ownership and start looking at menopause with a different attitude.

I'm hoping that, by now, you have at least shared a good laugh with me on this brief journey. A small part of this book was to encourage more joy. Another was a way to help as many of my sisters understand the complexities of menopause as possible. The most important thing that I would like for my sisters and brothers to take from me at this stage of a woman's life is that menopause is a time to be embraced.

Let's normalise this transition and change the dialogue from any negative connotations. Menopause is not an illness. It's a natural part of life. At this point in our lives, we are powerful, intelligent, amazing women. We have lived, loved, some have lost. We have overcome a multitude of hurdles and still got back on that horse. Remember that with age comes wisdom!

Walk fearlessly into your future with a renewed sense of confidence. Remember the dreams that you have yet to fulfil, the songs you are yet to sing. Make the changes that need to be done and don't wait until tomorrow. Now is the time to live your best life and find what works for you. Do what it takes to help yourself feel physically better. Do not be disheartened. Keep trying new things until you find your own cure.

Only then will we see a change in society, including our children and our men. Let's move on together from pain to power.

Until the next time, it has been my utmost pleasure, my Sisters, my Queens, and my Friends.

Now, if you are ready to make a start on embracing this new chapter, then turn the pages and enjoy a little gift from me to you.

The End

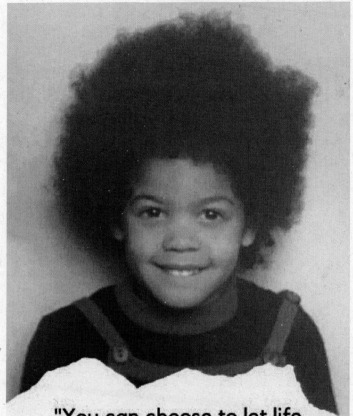

"You can choose to let life
make you, or break you.
Choose wisely"

JACQUELINE GOLDING

From Pause to Power

I didn't want to leave my queens without some simple, practical ideas to get you started on the quest to embrace this transition. The book will have highlighted the importance of supporting your sisters and seeking support for yourself.

I know for me, the jolt I needed was a little push from my children. I made some minor changes in my life which led to quick improvements. This further prompted me to address other things, but we all need a starting point, don't we?

We'll look at natural ways to reduce menopause symptoms through diet, exercise, mindfulness and creating safe physical spaces, so, please enjoy some little tips on how to create a nurturing environment and nurture your mind, body and spirit too!

Natural Ways to Reduce Symptoms of Menopause

As we have already established, I'm no doctor, so I can only speak from my own personal experiences and what I have heard from my sisters throughout this journey. I would always recommend consulting your GP, or someone who is qualified to give medical advice, on the best way to manage your symptoms. We all know by now just how unique each woman's menopausal transition is. Below are some tips and tricks that I've gathered along the way, mixed in with some advice from good old Doctor Google.

• Eating foods that are rich in Calcium and Vitamin D to reduce the risk of osteoporosis.

• Work on achieving and maintaining a healthy weight to help alleviate menopause symptoms and reduce the risk of heart disease.

• Eating plenty of fruit and vegetables as this will assist with weight maintenance and your intake of vitamins.

• Try to avoid trigger foods such as caffeine, alcohol and sugary or spicy foods to help reduce the triggering of hot flushes, night sweats and mood swings.

- Exercising regularly for improved energy and metabolism, healthier joints and bones, decreased stress and better sleep.

- Eating foods that are high in phytoestrogens like flax seeds and sesame seeds, beans like soybeans and edamame beans and dried fruits can help balance hormones. Phytoestrogens are naturally occurring plant compounds that can mimic the effects of oestrogen in the body.

- Drinking plenty of water can help with symptoms such as dryness and bloating.

- Reduce your intake of refined sugar and processed foods to reduce the feelings of tiredness and irritability.

- Don't skip meals as irregular eating can make certain symptoms of menopause worse and may even hinder weight loss efforts.

- Eating protein-rich foods regularly may prevent the loss of lean muscle, aid in weight loss and help regulate mood and sleep.

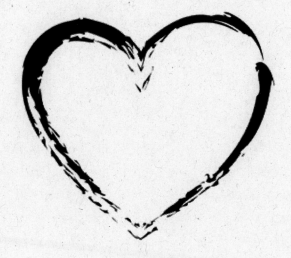

Connecting with Nature

Connecting with nature was a key element for me throughout my garden project. As hard as it was physically to keep going for months on end when there didn't seem to be an end in sight, the result we achieved was nothing short of magnificent. Watching each section of the garden be transformed and nurturing new and beautiful living things diminished any prior feeling I had about being worthless. The experience reaffirmed the knowledge I once had, that I am able to create amazing and mighty things, menopausal or not.

Nature sustains us and offers us all that we need to flourish. Nature can assist with balancing hormones and can even help to reduce some menopausal symptoms. Products of the soil help to keep our bodies healthy. Strolling on the seashore, in the forest, parks, or anyplace in nature re-energises us, quiets our psyche, sustains our spirits, and helps alleviate stress. Nature is key in nurturing the mind, body, and soul.

Angela, a colleague of mine, had suggested that I try 'forest bathing'. My immediate thought was that it sounded like some sort of strange open-air bathing experience in the woods but

Angela soon set me straight. Even though I am still yet to try forest bathing, I can confirm that it is cemented onto my bucket list.

Forest bathing (or shinrin-yoku) is a broad term meaning to immerse oneself in the therapeutic atmosphere of the forest with all of the senses. It doesn't need to be any more complicated than simply strolling through the woods or a park. The main distinction is that you set aside the effort to truly zero in on the natural world around you as opposed to strolling for exercise or to reach a destination. Picture yourself bathed in beams of daylight, soothed by birdsong echoing through the trees.

I am told that regular practice can help with reducing brain fog, improved temperament, memory and focus, lower stress levels, diminishing cortisol levels and lower blood pressure, as well as helping you to remain calm and strengthening your immune system.

Tips to remember when forest bathing:

1. Pick an area that you feel comfortable in. Consider the time of day you choose to bathe; you might prefer a time when there are fewer people around or a time when there is a bit more hustle and bustle.

2. Turn your phone to silent; a queen should enjoy her bath in peace.

3. Take as much time as you like - you may prefer to sit somewhere picturesque or meander throughout the woodlands. You may wish to be there for hours or even a quick ten-minute visit.

4. Use your senses. Feel the rough bark of tree trunks and delicate leaves and listen to the birdsong.

5. Try to relax and calm your mind. Breathing exercises are great to practise whilst forest bathing. They also help to focus your mind on your breathing and your surroundings.

Building a Sanctuary

I feel that it's important to have your own sanctuary, a safe and quiet space where you can practise mindfulness and allow yourself to relax. I built mine in my living room, in the form of a meditation corner. I filled it with an aromatherapy oil diffuser, an Alexa for music, candles and lots of nature-inspired art and objects.

Your sanctuary will be specific to you and it's important that wherever you create this space, you fill it with items, sounds and smells that you know will relax and calm your mind and body. For some, this may take shape as a hot bubble bath, surrounded with candles and accompanied by soothing music. For others, it may be a small 'me time' kit that can be carried around with you so that you are able to take a moment wherever you may be. Depending on the space you have available, you may choose to create a 'woman cave' of sorts, a whole room just for you. But remember that even in a small space, your sanctuary can still be created.

Easy Smoothies for Balancing Hormones

Smoothies are a great way to fuel your body and keep your blood sugar in check. By including four key elements in your smoothies, you can ensure that your body receives an elongated blood sugar curve which will reduce the chance of feeling sluggish and low in energy. These four key elements should also help to keep your hormones balanced but always remember to seek medical advice.

The four elements:

1. Protein
High-quality protein powder or collagen peptides can help with maintaining muscle mass, skin health, and joint pain.

2. Fat
Healthy fats such as any nut butter, coconut oil, hemp seeds, flax seeds, chia seeds, avocado, or MCT oil can help to provide energy, support cell growth, protect organs and can also help with hormone production.

3. Fibre

Sources of fibre can include chia seeds, acacia fibre, flax seeds, or even frozen cauliflower rice. Some studies have shown that fibre intake can reduce hot flushes in menopause.

4. Greens

Higher consumption of leafy greens and cruciferous vegetables (cabbage, cauliflower, kale, etc) can help in reducing overall menopausal symptoms, specifically physical symptoms.

Each of these three recipes include each key element and only take about ten minutes to prepare. Each recipe will make one serving of the smoothie so be sure to increase your measurements should you wish to make more than one.

Milk in each recipe can be replaced with any dairy-free milk such as almond milk, cashew milk, flax milk, walnut milk, coconut milk, etc.

Magnesium Magic Smoothie

A tasty mix of banana and nuts for when you need an energy boost.

- 1.5 cups of milk
- 1/2 large banana
- 1 tbsp of any nut butter
- 1 serving (scoop) protein powder or collagen peptides
- 1 tbsp cacao powder
- 2 tsp maca powder (optional)
- 2 tbsp chia seeds or acacia fiber
- 2 handfuls spinach leaves (about 2 cups)

Balancing Berry Smoothie

Use pomegranates, blueberries, blackberries, or raspberries for a high antioxidant count to help reduce oxidative stress.

- 1 1/4 cup of milk
- 2 tbsp chia seeds
- 1 serving (scoop) protein powder or collagen peptides
- 2/3 cup frozen cauliflower rice
- 2 handfuls spinach leaves
- 1/4 cup of any berries

Flush Flattener Smoothie

This green smoothie is loaded with vitamin C to help maintain healthy skin, blood vessels, bones and cartilage.

- 1 1/4 cup milk
- 1/3 cup diced courgette
- 1/4 large avocado
- 1/4 cup diced kiwi
- 3 tbsp hemp seeds
- 1 serving (scoop) protein powder or collagen peptides
- 2 handfuls chopped kale leave

Easy Yoga for Beginners

Over the years, I have tried various forms of exercise, from rollerblading to soca-cise, but I was yet to find something that I would commit to and be consistent with. Shortly after having my second child, in an effort to budge the baby weight, I decided to try pilates. I couldn't tell you that it made any kind of difference, but it was successful in relaxing me so much that I fell asleep mid-session and had to be woken up once the class had finished.

I had never really given much thought to yoga, except for observing that it looked incredibly difficult and, in my mind, could only be pulled off by a contortionist. Whilst on a work trip in Bulgaria with my PA last year, the opportunity to attend a yoga class had presented itself and, despite being a little worried about my own ability, I joined a beautiful group of ladies and decided to put myself to the test. I was pleasantly surprised. Not only did I survive the entire class, I actually enjoyed it. I felt completely relaxed and very pleased with myself. I now try to do yoga as often as possible because I can physically feel the benefits. Yoga can help to maintain your body's strength without overheating or over-exerting yourself.

Below I have listed five yoga poses that are easy to try and keep up with. They can be adapted for those of you with limited mobility and remember that some poses may not be suitable for everyone, so as with all things, you need to find what works for you.

1. Cat/cow pose

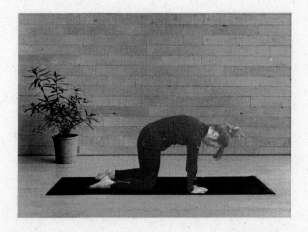

Start on your hands and knees. Line up your wrists directly beneath your shoulders. Line up your knees directly beneath your hips, and spread them apart at a distance equal to your inner hip-width. When you inhale, tuck your toes under and expand your upper chest forward, keeping your lower abdominals engaged and your lower spine in neutral. When you exhale, relax onto the tops of your feet, round your back through the lower spine, and completely relax your head. Work at an individual pace, coordinating your movements with your breaths.

2. Lunge pose

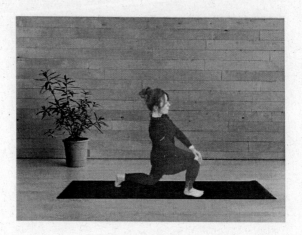

Start on your hands and knees. Step your right foot forward, in between your hands, so that the heel of your foot is lined up with the heels of both hands. Bring your torso into an upright position, and place your hands on your hips. Check to make sure your knee is directly over your ankle in a stacked position. Keep your shoulders relaxed and gaze straight ahead. Deepen the bend in your knee to feel the stretch in the hip flexor of your left leg. Open your chest and breathe deeply. Repeat on the other side.

3. Wide leg forward bend posture

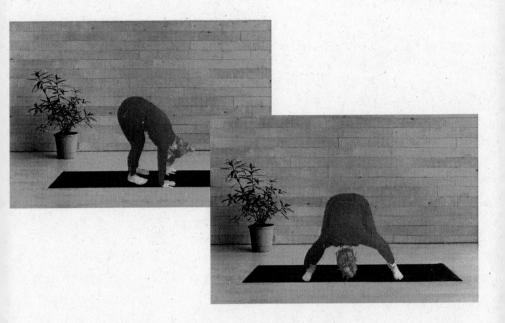

Stand with your legs a distance of one leg's length apart with toes facing forward. Line up your heels behind the wide parts of your feet. Fold forward at the hip crease, keeping your spine long, and hold on behind your ankles, keeping your head and neck long. Balance your weight through all four corners of your feet. Open through the chest and relax your shoulder blades onto the back.

4. Cobra pose

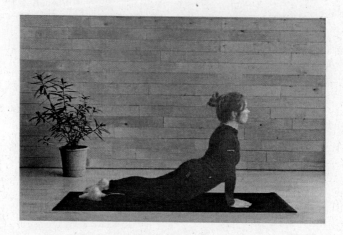

Lying on your belly, extend your legs directly behind you with your front thighs on the floor and all 10 toes pressing into the floor. Place your palms slightly forward of your shoulders, shoulder-width apart or slightly wider, forearms parallel, and fingers spread wide. Open through the front of your chest, lengthening and extending your spine. Activate your inner thighs and lift them toward the ceiling while relaxing your buttocks. Keep your neck in line with your spine and your gaze out in front on the floor.

5. Forward-facing hero pose

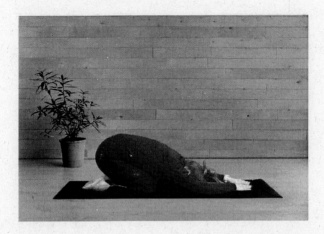

Place your knees mat-width apart and touch your big toes together with your heels apart. Sit on your heels. Lengthen your tailbone down toward the floor, keeping your spine long. Walk your hands forward until your spine is fully extended, and draw your shoulder blades onto your back. Keep your arms and hands shoulder-width apart. Relax your forehead onto the floor, keeping your neck long.

Mini Meditations

Although it is something I have done many times throughout my life, I won't pretend I'm a meditation guru, nor will I pretend that I found it easy to clear my mind and become a serene, peaceful goddess with just one minute's meditation. But what I will tell you is that after making a conscious effort to take time out of my day, I can definitely feel the benefit and meditation helps to relax my mind and reduce stress. It takes discipline and it doesn't happen overnight, but it's worth it.

I have included two quick and easy meditations that can help to ground you if you find yourself having a bit of a moment. Before beginning, make sure that you are somewhere comfortable and without too many distractions. Head to a quiet place or room where you can sit alone and allow yourself to take a couple of minutes. I also find that carrying some essential oils around, to use at times like these, can help you to relax and calm your mind.

Mini Meditations

Take a deep breath.

Breathing in through the nose.

Breathing out through the mouth.

Breathing in feeling the lungs expanding.

Breathing out feeling a sense of letting go.

Breathing in to feel the body getting fuller.

Breathing out to feel the release of any tension.

Breathing in feeling alive and awake.

Breathing out feeling muscles relaxing

Breathing in that sense of fullness.

Breathing out that unnecessary tension in the body and mind.

Mini Meditations

Start by drawing in a very deep breath from your stomach, filling your lungs from the bottom up.

Once you can't take in any more air, exhale by letting your breath out as slowly and controlled as possible.

Do a series of breaths where you breathe in, to the count of four, hold for four beats, and then exhale to the count of four and observe yourself passively breathing in and out.

Feel your breath going in and out through your nose and take note of how it feels as your lungs expand and contract.

Breathe in while saying, "I am," and then breathe out with a positive statement like "at peace."

Daily Affirmations

Daily affirmations are positive statements to encourage motivation and self-belief. Words can have such extreme power. Practised daily, affirmations help to challenge your lack of confidence, low self-esteem and enable you to overcome negative thoughts.

I have always recognised the power of using affirmations. I believe that repetition is the mother of skill. Just as negative thoughts can be incredibly damaging for your confidence and self-esteem, using positive daily affirmations can influence your unconscious mind and release you from worry and fear.

I have listed some affirmations below to give you some ideas and starting points but I would recommend using ones that feel specific to you or adapting them slightly for relevance.

Affirmations for low self-esteem:

I am good enough.

I am special to the world.

I am beautiful inside and out.

I love and accept myself.

Affirmations for confidence building and self-belief:

I am in full control of my life.

Every day I become more confident and powerful.

I know my potential and what it can give me.

There is so much power and strength within me.

Affirmations for finding love and a new relationship:

I deserve to be happy and loved.

I am worthy of love and deserve the best.

I am loving and lovable.

My heart and intuition will guide me

Affirmations for a new challenge in your life, i.e. new job or back to work:

I can handle any obstacles in my path.

I am braver and stronger than I realise.

I have huge potential and believe in myself.

I am competent, smart, and able.

Affirmations for physical challenges, i.e. weight loss and fitness:

I am totally focused on achieving my weight loss goal.

I control my weight with healthy eating.

I work out to feel good and fit.

My body is a gift, I treat it with love.

Affirmations for personal growth:

I continue to learn and grow.

The past doesn't define me.

I appreciate the lessons life has taught me.

There is no place in my life for disrespectful people.

Remember to trust yourself and keep it going – the best of you is yet to come.

About the Author

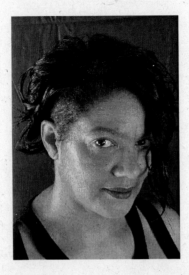

Jacqueline Golding is a first-time author of British/Irish and Jamaican heritage.

As a child, Jacqueline wrote constantly. Expressing herself through poetry, short stories and novels, Jacqueline used her writing to escape her painful childhood.

In adulthood, her life journey took her away from writing. She spent her career attending to the underprivileged members of society as a youth worker, family support worker, children's residential worker and independent skills advisor.

After meeting her menopause head-on, Jacqueline returned to her childhood love of writing. With a new sense of freedom and her usual compassion and empathy, she decided that her debut would encompass the voices of the voiceless.

This collective diary highlights not only Jacqueline's transition through womanhood, but also the journeys of women from around the world. Jacqueline's only rule was that each and every one of them told their truth.

The poignancy of this book shows that despite the challenges that the transition into menopause can bring, freedom is within reach for us all.

Website: https://www.menodiaries.co.uk/
Instagram: @jgoldingauthor
Facebook: @Jacquegolding

It always helps to support local authors, so please, if you enjoyed this novel, take a few minutes to leave a review on one or all of the following platforms:

Goodreads

Facebook

Stay blessed